Respiration

Respiration

The Breath of Life

By Dr. Peter Sebel,
    Dr. D. M. Stoddart,
    Dr. Richard E. Waldhorn,
    Dr. Carl S. Waldmann,
    Dr. Philip Whitfield

TORSTAR BOOKS
New York · Toronto

TORSTAR BOOKS INC.
300 E. 42nd Street
New York, NY 10017

THE HUMAN BODY
Respiration:
The Breath of Life

Publisher
Bruce Marshall

Art Director
John Bigg

Editor
Jinny Johnson

Art Editor
Mel Peterson

Text Editor
Gwen Rigby

Researchers: Pip Morgan, Jazz Wilson

Director of Picture Research
Zilda Tandy

Picture Researcher: Jessica Johnson

Artists:
Frank Kennard, Mike Courtney, Les Smith

Art Assistant: Arthur Brown

Cover Design
Moonink Communications

Cover Art: Paul Giovanopoulos

Director of Production: Barry Baker

Production Coordinator: Janice Storr

Business Director: Candy Lee

Planning Assistant: Avril Essery

International Sales: Barbara Anderson

In conjunction with this series Torstar Books offers an electronic digital thermometer which provides accurate body temperature readings in large liquid crystal numbers within 60 seconds.

For more information write to:
Torstar Books Inc.
300 E. 42nd Street
New York, NY 10017

Authors

Peter Sebel is a Senior Lecturer and Honorary Consultant in Anesthetics at the London Hospital Medical College. Previously he spent three years at the University of Amsterdam carrying out research programs in his special interest: the effects of anesthesia. He has published many articles in both European and American journals on the use of new drugs in anesthesia and their effects on the brain.

Mike Stoddart is a biologist and zoologist with particular interest in mammalian studies. He is the author of *The Ecology of Vertebrate Olfaction* and has also contributed to many other books on the natural sciences, including *The Animal Family* and *Rhythms of Life*.

Richard E. Waldhorn is Assistant Professor in the Department of Medicine, Pulmonary Disease Division, at the Georgetown University School of Medicine, Washington D.C. and Co-Medical Director of the Respiratory Therapy Department at Georgetown University Hospital. He is also Codirector of the Georgetown University Hospital Sleep Disorders Center. His special interests are clinical care medicine and sleep disorders and he is at present working on therapeutic approaches to sleep apnea.

Carl Waldmann is a Senior Registrar in anesthesia at the London Hospital. He served in the Air Force for five years as a physician, during which time he dealt with altitude-induced respiratory problems. His special interests include anesthesia in abnormal conditions (at altitude or at depth) and intensive care, and he is coauthor of *Intensive Therapy*. Dr. Waldmann has also contributed to medical journals on the subject of anesthesia.

Philip Whitfield is a biologist and zoologist with a wide range of interests. He has written and contributed to many books, including *The Animal Family*, *Jungles*, *Rhythms of Life* and *The Biology of Parasitism*.

Series Consultants

Donald M. Engelman is a Professor of Molecular Biophysics and Biochemistry and Professor of Biology at Yale. He has pioneered new methods for understanding cell membranes and ribosomes, and has also worked on the problem of atherosclerosis. He has published widely in professional and lay journals and lectured at many universities and international conferences.

Stanley Joel Reiser is Professor of Humanities and Technology in Health Care at the University of Texas Health Center in Houston. He is author of *Medicine and the Reign of Technology*; coeditor of *Ethics in Medicine: Historical Perspectives and Contemporary Concerns*; and coeditor of the anthology *The Machine at the Bedside*.

Harold C. Slavkin, Professor of Biochemistry at the University of Southern California, directs the Graduate Program in Craniofacial Biology and also serves as Chief of the Laboratory for Developmental Biology in the University's Gerontology Center.

Lewis Thomas is Chancellor of the Memorial Sloan-Kettering Cancer Center in New York City and University Professor at the State University of New York, Stony Brook. A member of the National Academy of Sciences, Dr. Thomas has served on advisory councils of the National Institutes of Health.

Consultants for Respiration

Edward R. McFadden is the Argyl J. Beams Professor of Medicine at the Case Western Reserve University School of Medicine, and Physician and Director of the Asthma and Allergic Disease Center at University Hospitals, Cleveland, Ohio. He has held Visiting Professorships at a number of university medical schools including Yale, Duke and Johns Hopkins. A specialist in pulmonary medicine, his major research interests include the mechanics of respiration and asthma, and he has served on a number of research committees investigating lung function and disease. He has contributed to many books, including the American Physiology Society *Handbook of Physiology* and *Harrison's Principles of Internal Medicine*.

Edward C. Rosenow, III is Professor of Medicine at the Mayo Medical School, Rochester, Minnesota and Program Director of the Internal Medicine Residency Program at the Mayo Clinic. He is also a member of the Pulmonary Subspecialty Board of the American Board of Internal Medicine. Dr. Rosenow is particularly interested in the effects of drugs on lung function and is editor of the journal *Seminars on Respiratory Medicine*, the most comprehensive review of drug-induced pulmonary disease.

©Torstar Books Inc. 1985

Library of Congress Cataloging in Publication Data
Main entry under title:

Respiration, the breath of life.

Includes index.
1. Respiration. 2. Respiratory organs. 3. Respiratory organs—Diseases. I. Sebel, Peter. [DNLM: 1. Respiration. 2. Respiratory System. 3. Respiratory Tract Diseases. WF 102 R4345] QP121.R44 1985 612'.2 85-2529

ISBN 0-920269-22-2 (The Human Body series)
ISBN 0-920269-41-9 (Respiration)
ISBN 0-920269-42-7 (leatherbound)
ISBN 0-920269-43-5 (school ed.)

20 19 18 17 16 15 14 13 12 11
10 9 8 7 6 5 4 3 2 1

Contents

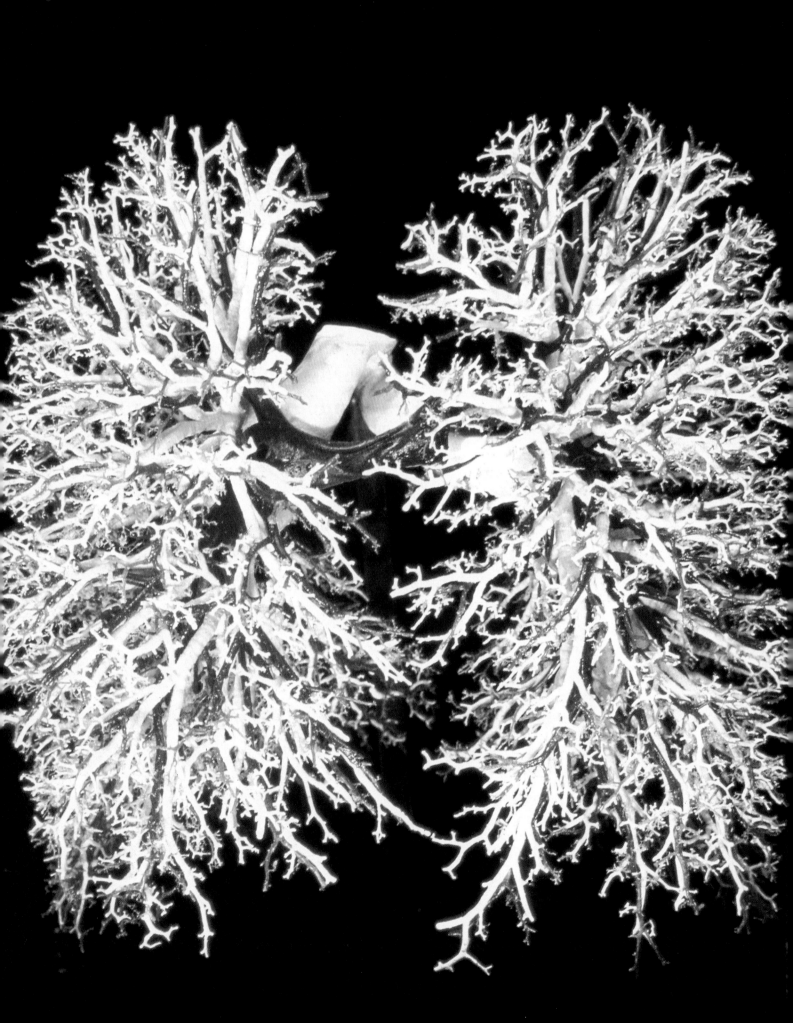

Introduction:

A Life-giving System

Inside the human lungs is a complex system of branching airways, here seen as a resin cast. The single trachea, or windpipe, divides into two bronchi, one of which passes into each lung. Each bronchus branches many times to produce a treelike structure of finer and finer air tunnels. The smallest tubes, the bronchioles, of which there are over 260,000, terminate in millions of alveoli — the tiny air spaces where gas exchange with the blood takes place. In this cast, the bronchial passages are white and the pulmonary artery and veins, red.

A newborn baby takes its first breath of life — the breath that signals the start of independent existence. With that first inrush of air, a near-miraculous series of physiological alterations to the baby's blood vessels and lungs is set in motion to convert it from dependence on the life-supporting placenta to air-breathing autonomy. A marathon runner, shoulders and chest heaving with each painful breath, staggers across the finishing line three hours and twenty-six miles after he began running. An Andean miner works daily at an altitude at which a lowlander, unaccustomed to conditions of low atmospheric pressure, would soon be gasping after the least activity.

Each of these vignettes of human activity underlines the extraordinary adaptability of human respiration. A breath in, a breath out, fourteen or so times every minute, seems a simple and unexceptional formula on which to base a life-giving system of ventilation and respiration. This simplicity is deceptive, however, and breathing is instantly and amazingly responsive to the most subtle changes in mood, level of alertness or activity.

Without any conscious willing for change, emotion, as well as exertion, will switch on marked shifts in a pattern of breathing. Apprehension induces a racing of the pulse and faster, shallower breathing. Fear can cause a sharp intake of breath and then tense breathholding. No physical exertion has occurred, but a changed emotional state is as potent a stimulus to the controlling system for breathing as the first few steps in a race.

The Greeks believed that air — pneuma — was a thing of the spirit, an entity that man needed to charge his body with vitality. Today's physiologists have a more functional concept of the workings of the lungs. But, when considering the imperative bonds between breathing and life, it is tempting to conclude that the Greek view encapsulated a vibrant and central truth.

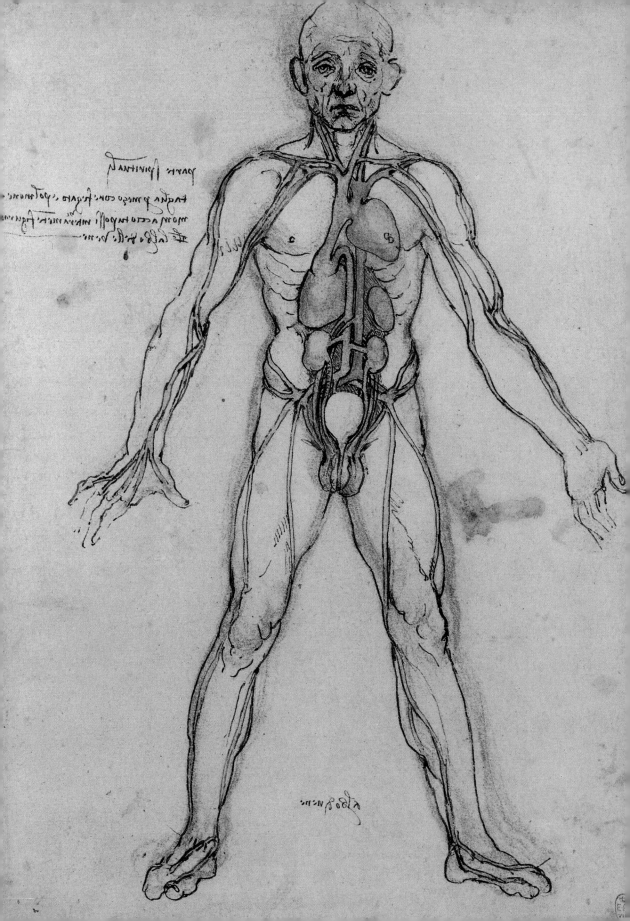

Chapter 1

The Vital Spirit

Breathing equals living. Except in the deepest phases of sleep or unconsciousness, the chest and abdominal movements of human respiration are a constant, reiterated reassurance that life and health continue. As this relationship between breathing and vitality follows from the simplest direct observation, it must have been part of the human world view for hundreds of thousands of years. It is a correlation described in verse, prose, sagas, folklore and holy books in a multitude of ways — some direct, some fanciful — but always pointing to the same inevitable conclusion: if you breathe you live, and if you live you breathe.

The Holy Bible makes the link in its description of man's creation:

> And the Lord God formed man of the dust of the ground and breathed into his nostrils the breath of life; and man became a living soul.
>
> Genesis 2, 7

According to Genesis, man's body is first constructed, then life is added by the acquisition of holy breath. This relationship might almost be a parable of another self-evident truth — every independent human life begins with a baby's first breath. As is appropriate, life outside the womb is signaled by that most moving of events — the primal cry and breath of the newborn. Before there was any real knowledge of fetal development, it would have been reasonable to assume that a baby was physically constructed within its mother and then acquired life at the moment of birth, with its first breath. From that starting point, with breath being intimately connected with the beginning of every ordinary human life, it is a natural extrapolation to assert that God gave humankind life by means of a holy, exogenous breath.

The life-breath dualism occurs again and again in literature. The nineteenth-century poet John Keats, in Book 1 of *Endymion*, produced a marvelous

An anatomical drawing of a man, showing heart, lungs and main arteries, typifies Leonardo da Vinci's interest in the structure of the human body. Part of a series of studies probably made to illustrate anatomical theories, the drawing dates from about 1504–06 and shows an accuracy and perception far superior to anything preceding it. The function of those organs so skillfully depicted was, however, to remain a mystery for many more years to come.

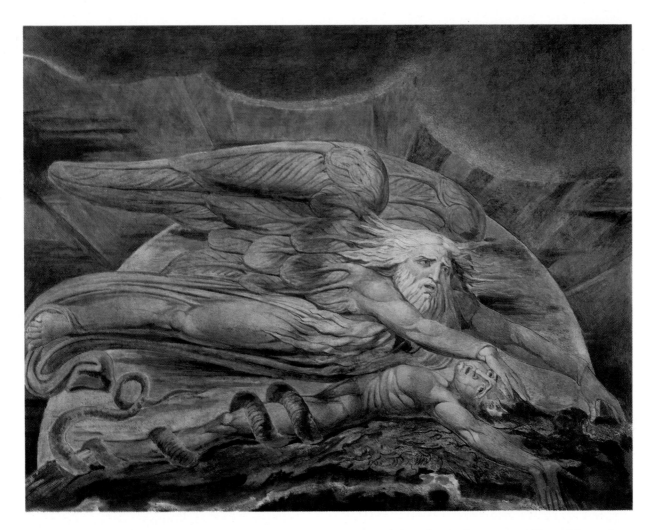

encapsulation of the meaning of beauty:

> A thing of beauty is a joy forever ...

and then continues with a calm evocation of the way in which light breathing signals a particular, tranquil state of body and mind:

> Its loveliness increases: it will never
> Pass into nothingness; but still will keep
> A bower quiet for us, and a sleep
> Full of sweet dreams, and health, and quiet
>   breathing.

Alfred, Lord Tennyson, in *The Two Voices* speaks more starkly of the inner knowledge of the irreducible conjunction between the breathing of air and continued earthly existence:

> Whatever crazy sorrow saith,
> No life that breathes with human breath
> Has ever truly longed for death.

Breathing, mainly generated and controlled by unconscious mechanisms, is such an accustomed part of life that few people give it a moment's consideration in a normal day. We only become aware of the physical process of breathing when something impairs the smooth automatic cycle of inspiration and expiration that underlies every minute of our lives. Increased exertion — jogging, climbing, swimming or cycling — makes additional demands for more oxygen, and suddenly we are conscious of an unaccustomed urgency in the pattern and depth of our breaths. Temporary cessation of breathing, as in a long, unassisted dive, makes the first gasp of air on breaking through the water surface a savored joy. Respiratory disease can also put the need to breathe actively and well into sharp, and sometimes painful, focus.

Such everyday factors point to the vital role of breathing and its links with levels of activity. Of themselves, however, they reveal nothing of the reasons behind our need to breathe. Why on earth should the human body be built around a design plan which requires it to take in and then push out the gaseous atmosphere that surrounds it? Why on earth is perhaps an apt way of posing the question, because ultimately the answer is to be sought in the physical evolution of planet Earth over four and a half billion years. The particular development of both the Earth's crust and its atmosphere provide the template upon which our system of respiration was molded.

Within a billion years, at the most, of the establishment of Earth as an individually distinct planet, its watery surface was dramatically transformed by the presence of life. Embedded in rock sediments some three and a half billion years old are microfossils of simple, single-celled, probably bacterialike organisms of the organizational type classified as prokaryotic. For about another two billion years, these lifeforms dominated the globe — a globe which almost all evidence suggests had an atmosphere devoid of oxygen. Carbon dioxide was present, as was water vapor and nitrogen, but the air of the planet was without what to us is its most significant component. All the early prokaryotic lifeforms must have been anaerobes, that is, organisms that can carry out all their metabolic functions, including the internal provision of usable energy, without oxygen.

The Atmosphere Changes

About one and a half billion years ago, the primeval atmosphere began to alter. The change was a deceptively simple one: oxygen began to appear in the atmosphere in increasing quantities, prompting the evolution of more complex cell types and, subsequently, complex multicellular organisms. Most research workers in this field believe that the atmospheric change was the work of living rather than nonliving agencies for it is likely that it was achieved by blue-green algae.

Blue-green algae developing at around this geological moment in Earth's history solved the biochemical puzzle of using water (H_2O) as a hydrogen source in the process of photosynthesis, by which lifeforms construct complex organic molecules from simple inorganic ones. More primitive photosynthetic prokaryotes had used sources such as hydrogen sulphide (H_2S), but, utilizing water, sunlight energy and carbon dioxide in their new form of photosynthesis, the blue-green algae could efficiently construct all the vital organic molecules that a cell needs. They became the dominant lifeform on planet Earth and in so doing they polluted it in a remarkable way. By using water

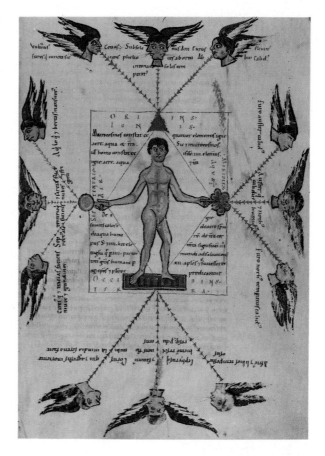

An illustration from a twelfth-century manuscript reflects the belief, current at the time, that man, the microcosm, was at the center of the world and the basic elements, the macrocosm.

11

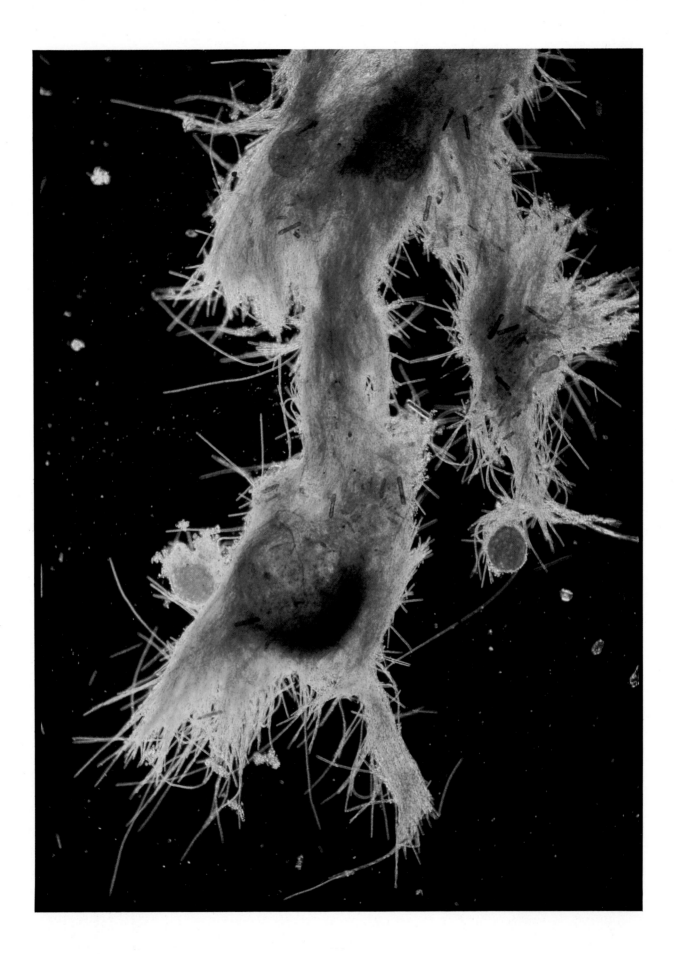

Blue-green algae (left) are among the most primitive cells that can photosynthesize. Their ancestors probably transformed the Earth's atmosphere from an anaerobic gas mixture to one containing oxygen.

Symbols of life, the heart and lungs were the organs torn out during the ritual human sacrifices performed by the Aztecs of Central America. These vital parts of the body were offered in homage to the gods.

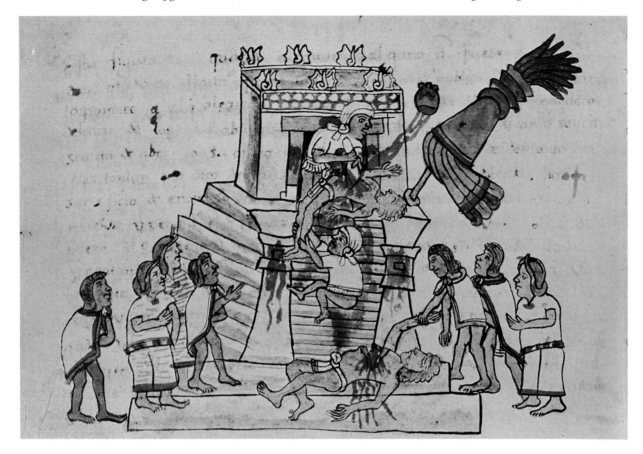

as a photosynthetic hydrogen source they gave off oxygen (the O in H_2O) as a waste product. That waste product transformed the atmosphere and the course of Earthly evolution.

With increasing concentrations of oxygen in the atmosphere, organisms developed new biochemical and metabolic strategies to cope with the novel situation. Oxygen can be a somewhat toxic molecule within cells, and some of these strategies involved new protective methods against this toxicity. Most important, though, organisms began to employ oxygen-using methods of generating available energy within their cells: a set of mechanisms together described as oxidative internal respiration. Within cell organelles, known as mitochondria, organic "fuels," ultimately derived from sugars such as glucose, "burned" with oxygen in a series of chemical steps controlled by biochemical catalysts or enzymes. This oxidation process supplied energy-rich compounds to drive

all the activities of the cell. Man and all the fifty thousand or so species of vertebrate animals existing on earth are among the most recently evolved of such oxygen-dependent, or aerobic, organisms.

Blue-green algae still exist; they may form, for instance, a scum of green slime around the edge of a muddy pond. Without the photosynthesis of the ancestors of that slime, the Earth as we know it would not have evolved.

Our oxygen-utilizing lungs are closely linked with the pumping heart and blood circulation. Like breathing movements, both the constant beat of the heart and the rhythm of the pulse have been regarded as "signs of life" from antiquity; all cultures have made the correlation between the beating heart and continuing life. Less obvious, though, and only fully grasped in historically recent times, has been the direct functional interrelationship between blood flow and breath.

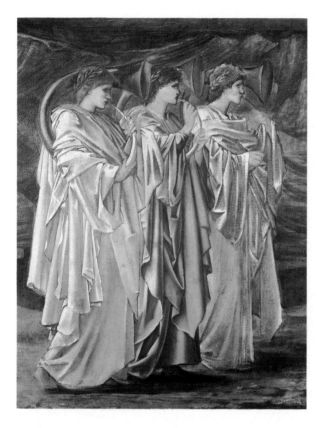

Via the channels of wind instruments, breath produces music. Graceful heralds here sound their horns in a painting, Challenge in the Wilderness, *by Sir Edward Burne-Jones (1838–98).*

The realization that it is blood which acts as the transport system for oxygen breathed in from the air, and for carbon dioxide that must be breathed out, is one that could only follow a reasonably sophisticated grasp of human physiology.

The Vital Bond

Breath and heartbeat are often joined in powerful poetic images. It is as though the potency of the two processes as metaphors for the vitality of human existence forces an understanding of their connection beyond the necessity of scientific proof.

William Wordsworth (1770–1850) in his poem, *Lines composed a few miles above Tintern Abbey*, talked of the mood of repose and keen responsiveness in which enlightenment dawns.

> . . . the breath of this corporeal frame
> And even the motion of our human blood
> Almost suspended, we are laid asleep
> In body, and become a living soul.

In describing that enviable configuration of mind and body, he seems to reveal instinctive knowledge of the linked functions of heart and lungs.

A little later, George Meredith (1828–1909) in *Hymn to Colour* suggests even more profound insight into the bond between blood and breath:

> Shall man into the mystery of breath
> From his quick beating pulse a pathway spy?
> Or learn the secret of the shrouded death,
> By lifting up the lid of a white eye?

What Meredith described as "the mystery of breath" — the mechanisms of human breathing and the physiological roles of the lung — has been center stage in many of the key periods of the development of scientific and medical knowledge. The process of respiration became a battleground over the centuries for rival and successive concepts concerning its functioning. These concepts rarely touched solely on the lungs as such; more often the historical ideas concerning respiration were part of integrated perceptions of the functioning of the human body as a whole. In other instances, development of central ideas in nonmedical scientific areas was dependent on investigations being made concerning the workings of the lungs.

In the latter half of the twentieth century, it might appear as though scientists have a wholly satisfactory understanding of the nature and implications of respiration. The structure of the two lungs within the chest cavity, surrounded externally by a flattened pleural sac, is known. The tubes or ducts — bronchioles, bronchi and trachea — that connect the substance of the lungs to the air cavity of the mouth and through which air can pass to the real working areas of the lungs, are fully described. These working areas are known to consist of alveoli, myriad tiny, rounded air spaces where air is brought into close proximity to blood in capillaries that enmesh each alveolus.

It is also known that across an amazingly narrow tissue barrier in each alveolus, oxygen diffuses into the capillary bed and becomes attached to hemoglobin molecules for subsequent transport around the body. And it is known that the gaseous bodily waste product carbon dioxide diffuses in the opposite direction, to be removed from the body in exhaled air. The muscle movements that enable us to take in each breath have been mapped, and the elastic tissue in each lung, whose contraction makes expiration possible, investigated. A clearer picture exists of the nervous and hormonal control systems that pattern our breathing, and the inventory of facts known about the lungs seems endless.

Turning Points in Science

But such moments in scientific development, when it appears that all the facts are tidily stored away, are exactly the times when a new idea, an original experiment, a moment of serendipidity in a single worker's observations can blow up the whole neat assemblage of supposedly accepted truths. At the end of the nineteenth century, for example, it must have seemed that chemistry and physics were in a reasonably organized, carefully pigeonholed state. Then in a three-year period, from 1905 to 1907, a Technical Expert (Second Class), working in the Patent Office in Berne, Switzerland, published some papers, and the edifice began to crumble. His name was Albert Einstein.

Such instances do not mean that the basic understanding of lung function and respiratory physiology is in imminent danger of being undermined by a single new discovery. They should merely serve as a reminder that every question answered about the lungs poses another

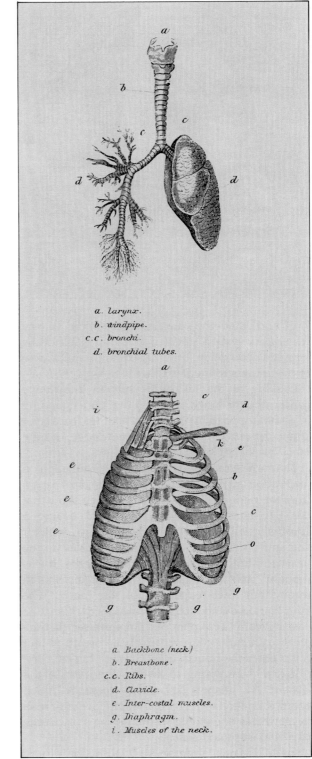

a. larynx.
b. windpipe.
c.c. bronchi.
d. bronchial tubes.

a. Backbone (neck)
b. Breastbone.
c.c. Ribs.
d. Clavicle.
e. Inter-costal muscles.
g. Diaphragm.
i. Muscles of the neck.

Empedocles, a Greek philosopher, poet and physician of the fifth century B.C., (below right) believed that all matter was composed of four basic elements: earth, fire, water and air (below left). Everything resulted from the combination or separation of these four. A balance of the elements, and the linked four humors, within the human body resulted in good health, an imbalance, bad health.

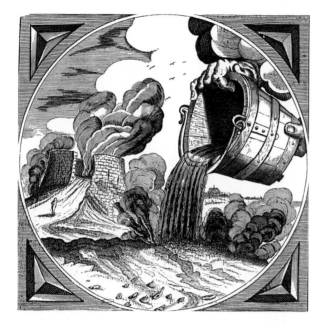

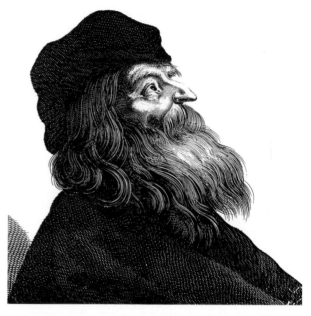

two and that the present conception of the respiratory system, detailed though it is, is not the ultimate description. Such descriptions are capable of continuous refinement.

Looking at the history of human knowledge concerning the lungs, it is clear that understanding of respiratory activity has been built up from layer after layer of accumulated new knowledge, despite many backward steps and blind alleys.

The earliest recorded examples of information on respiration are those in the Egyptian medical papyri from the period 2750 to 2625 B.C., which show that the Egyptians regarded air itself as having a spiritual quality. Breathing, in their view, took air and spirit in through the nostrils and then via the heart and lungs. From these primal organs, it was thought that the vital spirit was distributed throughout the remainder of the body. The Egyptians knew about the air-filled Eustachian tube passing from ear to pharynx and surmised that the breath of death, counterpart of the breath of life, could enter the human body through the left ear.

It would be wrong to dismiss the ideas of the ancient Egyptians, since they contain much genuine understanding. For life spirit of the air read oxygen, and one whole section of the story in the papyri makes good sense.

In the half millenium beginning at about 500 B.C.

the idea of the spirit-imbued nature of air surfaces again, with the philosophy and science of the Greeks and Romans.

Pneuma — Vital Spirit

Central to nearly all Greek philosophical thought throughout this period was the idea that the insubstantial, yet vital, essence within all things was "pneuma." Variously rendered in modern translations as spirit, breath or air, pneuma has passed into modern English in words such as pneumatic. No literal equality should be assumed, however, between the modern mechanistic conception of air as a mixture of gases and the Greek idea: pneuma was conceived as a crucial and all-pervading influence that was essential for life.

Empedocles, a Greek physician and philosopher who lived from about 495 to 435 B.C., put this concept, with three other elements, into a formal framework. The four, which he regarded as the basis of all matter, were earth, fire, water and air, or pneuma; he also postulated that there was a symmetrically similar set of four qualities: dry, hot, wet and cold. When elements and qualities were combined, the four vital humors of the body were generated, and a strange foursome they are to modern eyes: blood, phlegm, yellow bile and black bile. One explanation for disease at this time was

16

that it resulted from an imbalance of these humors.

Empedocles also had views on the purpose of human respiration: he thought that breathing in and out served to cool the heart and blood. Blood itself was felt to carry ''innate heat'' from the heart to all the other regions of the body.

The Animating Spirit

Fifty years after the death of Empedocles, another Greek philosopher was born whose impact on later generations was very much greater. Aristotle (384–322 B.C.) was strongly influenced by the ideas of Empedocles and subscribed to the element-quality-humor theories. But, in addition, he was a vitalist, convinced that living things could not be explained completely by physical, mechanistic and deterministic causes. To incorporate this aspect into the description of the nature of things, he invoked the existence of an animating spirit or ''psyche,'' which was the differentiating principle between living and inanimate objects. Like pneuma, psyche has been thoroughly integrated into modern English in words such as psychology.

After Aristotle, there is a jump of some four hundred years until the next great corpus of medically related knowledge focusing specifically on respiratory physiology: the copious writings of Galen (c. A.D. 130–199).

Galen was born in Pergamum, in eastern Turkey, and his father was a mathematician and architect. Galen studied medicine, first in his home town, then in Smyrna, Corinth and Alexandria. He became surgeon to the gladiators at Pergamum — a post which must have given him ample opportunities to observe internal aspects of human anatomy — and then traveled to Rome, where he was soon renowned as a physician, anatomist, author and teacher.

Galen's literary output, particularly of anatomical texts, was staggering: over one hundred, often massive, separate works are still in existence today. He provided a basic and highly detailed program of stages for the dissection of monkeys or human cadavers that was the orthodox medical training for almost fifteen hundred years — an extraordinary monument to the energy and enterprise of a single human being. William Harvey, who in the seventeenth century destroyed the central aspects

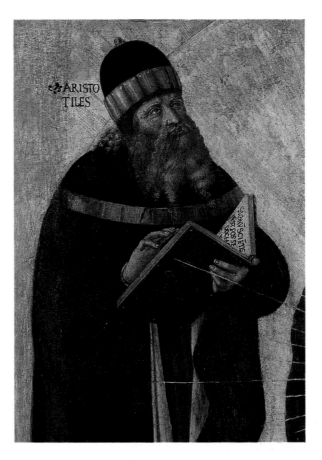

Philosopher, logician and scientist, Aristotle believed that the heart was the body's most important organ and that it generated essential warmth, without which other physical functions could not operate. He saw the lungs simply as a cooling system to control this heat, with inspiration of breath being stimulated by the buildup of heat in the heart.

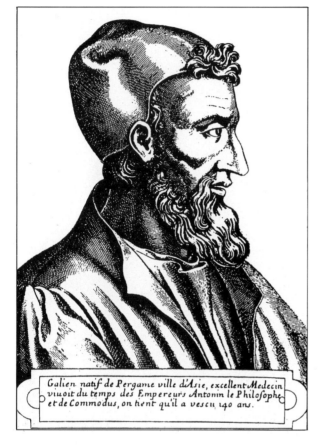

Galien natif de Pergame ville d'Asie, excellent Medecin vivoit du temps des Empereurs Antonin le Philosophe et de Commodus, on tient qu'il a vescu 140 ans.

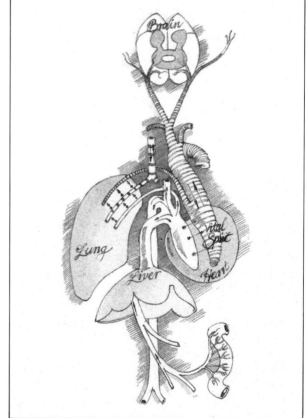

of Galen's physiological dogma, studied dissection for two years at the University of Padua, using the Galenic program of dissection drawn up fourteen hundred and fifty years before.

Galen's physiology generally, and his thoughts on respiration, were based partly on his direct, often anatomical, observations and partly on principles of a more philosophical nature which were regarded as almost self-evident at the time. It was believed that pneuma, or air, drawn into the human body by respiration, had to be adapted in three ways by the organs and processes of the body. These were linked to the three grades of activity of man, who was the highest form of living matter, growth, movement and thought. In its first transformation, air was changed to "natural spirit," linked with growth processes. The second change engendered "vital spirit," which itself was the mainspring of human passions; and in the third, pneuma, or air, was altered into "animal spirit"

(from the Greek *anima*, or soul), which could provoke thought.

Galen constructed a framework of physiological ideas that linked these supposed changes to particular organ systems. Almost all the ideas are misguided to a modern physiologist, but they fitted the philosophical views of Galen's time perfectly. Galen believed blood was formed in the liver from ingested food substances transported from the intestines by the portal veins. In the liver, the blood gained natural spirit and was then passed to the right ventricle of the heart. From here, some of the blood went through the pulmonary artery to sustain the lungs and to lose impurities in exhaled air. Another portion of the purified blood passed through the muscular wall (septum) between right and left ventricles via "invisible pores." In the large left ventricle, the blood was met by pneuma picked up from inspired air in the lungs and was transported from there by the pulmonary veins.

Anatomy was a popular subject of
study in the early eighteenth
century. Although demonstrations to
students improved knowledge of the
structure of the lungs, their function
was understood only later.

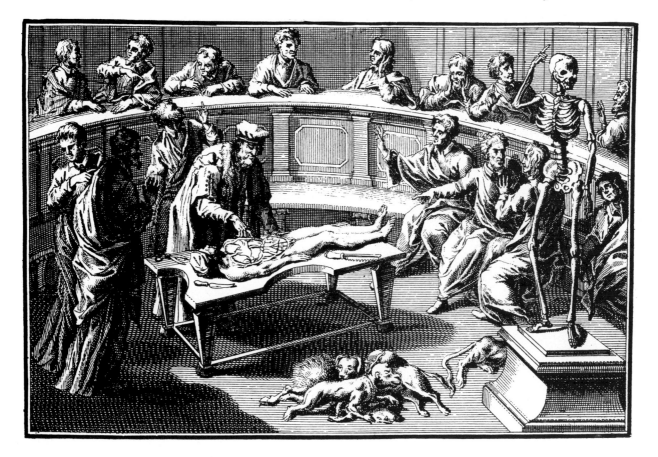

This mixing gave the blood the quality of "vital spirit," which could be transferred to all parts of the body through the main arteries. The arteries taking blood to the brain were finally supposed to transform some blood into "animal spirit" in a network of fine blood vessels at the base of the brain. The "animal spirit" passed to all other parts of the body along the nerves emanating from the brain.

The Passage of Blood

Thus Galen built up his masterly construction of internally flawed logic. During the Dark Ages, after the fall of the Roman Empire, his teachings and those of Aristotle were kept alive mainly in Arabic translations, while in Europe scientific and medical enquiry virtually ceased. During those bleak years, and until the sixteenth century, it was an Arabian scholar who made a single gigantic improvement on Galen's mixture of physiological impossibilities.

Ibn al-Nafis (1210–88), Dean of the Mansoury Hospital in Cairo, Egypt, forcefully put forward the proposition that, far from passing through "invisible pores" in the interventricular septum, blood actually passed from the right to the left ventricle of the heart via the lungs. In his *Commentary on the Anatomy of Avicenna*, he argued, correctly, that blood passed from the heart to the lungs along the pulmonary arteries and returned to it via the pulmonary veins. He was also perfectly justified in surmising that there must be blood vessel connections between the pulmonary arteries and veins within the substance of the lungs — connections now known to be the alveolar-capillary system.

Ibn al-Nafis is thought to have died peacefully at the age of sixty-eight, a respected member of his community. The independent rediscovery of the basic incompatibility between Galenic orthodoxy and the realities of the body by Renaissance theologian and physician Miguel Servetus brought him a more violent, untimely death. Born in 1509,

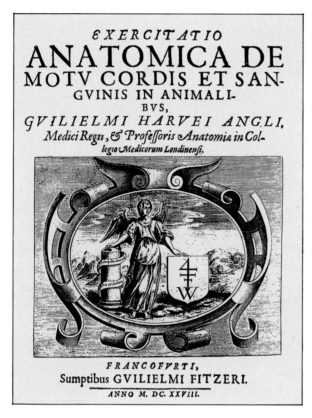

In 1628, English physician William Harvey published his masterpiece On the Motion of the Heart and Blood in Animals, *once and for all overthrowing Galenic theories. By his experiments on animals, Harvey demonstrated what Galen had not understood: that blood, pumped by the heart, circulates in a closed system. Although Harvey did little work on respiration itself, his clarification of the functions of the heart paved the way for later dramatic revelations of the linked functions of the heart and lungs.*

Servetus believed that anatomical studies could lead man to a better understanding of God's design. He reached correct conclusions about pulmonary blood flow and even noted the increased reddening of the blood after its passage through the lungs. (This change is caused by the conversion of the oxygen-carrying protein hemoglobin into its oxygen-rich, or oxidized oxyhemoglobin, form.) These and other remarkable insights set out in his book *Christianismi Restitutio* were considered heretical by both the Catholic Church and the Calvinists, as was his theological position. In 1553, at the age of forty-four, the percipient Servetus was burned at the stake in Geneva at the express order of John Calvin.

Religiously inspired suppression of scientific discoveries was not the only cause for the disorderly, "two steps forward, one step back" fashion in which knowledge of respiration accumulated during the sixteenth, seventeenth and eighteenth centuries. Even if findings were published, no efficient means existed for the widespread dissemination of scientific literature. As a result, discoveries made in one country could be unheard of decades, or even a century, later in another.

This was a period of independent rediscoveries of what, with the advantage of historical hindsight, can be seen to be single conclusions. The true route by which blood passes from the right to the left side of the heart — via the lungs — was discovered by Ibn al-Nafis in the thirteenth century and Miguel Servetus in the middle of the sixteenth. Yet another worker, Realdus Columbus (1516–59), who succeeded the anatomist Vesalius as Professor of Anatomy at Padua, came to an identical, but independent, conclusion around the same time. Some historians credit a third Renaissance worker with the discovery: Andreas Caesalpinus (1519–1603), who held the Chair of Medicine and Botany in the University of Pisa.

Many of the problems that impeded a rational explanation of the linked functions of heart and lungs from the time of Galen onward arose from the fact that the circulation of the blood was still unsuspected. It was known, of course, that blood moved in blood vessels — any soldier seeing blood spurt from a severed artery of a wounded man could have come to that conclusion. But in Galen's orthodoxy, it was believed that the blood surged around in a tidal-flow fashion, moving first in one direction, then in another.

The Connecting Systems

In the seventeenth century, this blockage to progress was removed by the English physician William Harvey (1578–1657). Harvey studied first at the University of Cambridge, then spent two significant years in Padua at the university before returning to London to work at the College of Physicians. In his epoch-making book *On the Motion of the Heart and Blood in Animals*, published in 1628, he proved conclusively that the heart was the pump in a continuous circulation system of blood. Suddenly the pulmonary and body circulation systems, driven by the two sides of the heart, became understandable as one interconnected moving stream of blood.

In 1661, the Italian scientist Marcello Malpighi (1628–94), by his microscope investigations, was able to extend the advance made by Harvey. He found the missing link in the pulmonary circulation — the capillary network that ultimately makes the pulmonary arteries and veins confluent with one another within the lungs. For his experiments, Malpighi used frog lungs; easy to obtain and small in size, they were simpler to work with and understand microscopically than the lungs of a human or any large mammal. By this means, Malpighi was able to demonstrate to the scientific world the structure of the alveoli and alveolar capillaries, where gas exchange takes place.

Between the publication of Harvey's important book in 1628 and the end of the century, advances on a number of fronts were being made at England's Oxford University that should have signaled an accelerating rate of understanding of respiratory physiology. Robert Boyle (1627–91), Robert Hooke (1635–1703), Richard Lower (1631–91) and John Mayow (1643–79) all made startling and interconnected discoveries in this field. It was shown that a component in air, crucial for an animal's survival, was being taken in by respiration; that blood passing through the lungs changed color, becoming redder rather than blue because of the uptake of part of the air by the blood;

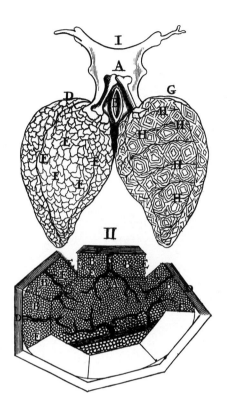

Generally considered one of the fathers of microscopy, Italian scientist Marcello Malpighi provided essential clues in the unraveling of the mystery of respiration. By his microscope observations of frog lungs, he discovered the existence of the alveoli (where gas exchange takes place) and the capillaries, without fully understanding their function. Above is his engraving of the cardiovascular system of the frog and a detail of its lung, showing the capillaries.

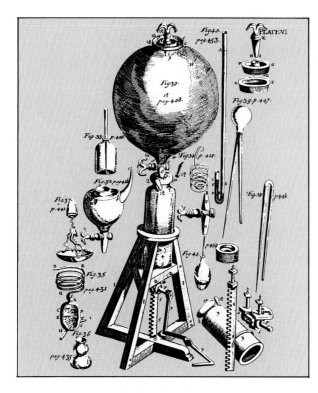

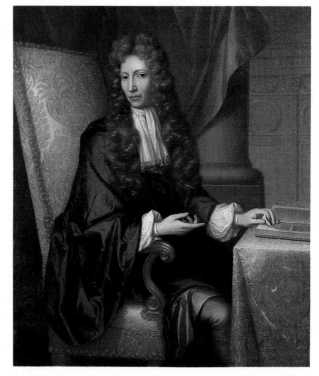

With another scientist, Robert Hooke, Boyle performed experiments to find the length of time an animal could survive in a closed vessel. They constructed an air pump (above) and found that if the pressure in the container was reduced, the animal's period of survival was shortened, but if they compressed the air, it lived longer. Their work proved that there was something in the air essential to every animal's survival.

and that the air component involved in these processes was also the part essential for the burning of any substance in air. Without identifying oxygen, these workers had reached several central and essentially correct conclusions about it and its role in respiration and combustion.

Unfortunately, this progress was bogged down in the mire of a contradictory and erroneous theory centered on the concept of phlogiston. Originally put forward by Georg Ernst Stahl (1660–1734), this theory suggested that when substances burned they lost phlogiston, rather than taking anything from the air. This almost complete inversion of the truth (substances *gain* oxygen when they burn in air) stifled development in respiration studies until Joseph Priestley (1733–1804), in Britain and then Pennsylvania, and Antoine Lavoisier (1743–94), in France, broke the logjam. Between them they clearly showed the true identity of atmospheric oxygen, its function as the vital gas in inspired air, and its role in energy production in the body, linked with the removal of carbon dioxide in exhaled air. At last, the mystery of respiration was beginning to be unraveled.

Joseph Priestley

Discoverer of Pure Air

A laundry tub, clay tobacco pipes, and wine and beer glasses were some of the utensils Joseph Priestley employed in his first experiments into the chemistry of gases.

Priestley was born in 1733 in Yorkshire, England, the son of Calvinist parents. As a boy he read widely and was an avid learner of languages, logic and philosophy. In 1752, he entered the Dissenting Academy — a school started by Nonconformists — where he studied theology with some of the best teachers in the land. After graduating, he began preaching, first in Suffolk then in Cheshire, where he opened a day school. A pioneer in education, Priestley began to feel a growing interest in science.

In 1762, Priestley was ordained a Dissenting Minister, but he was also busy teaching at a new Dissenting Academy and developing new courses for students, based on industry and commerce. On becoming Minister of the Mill Hill Chapel in Leeds, in 1767, he found himself living next to a brewery, where the effervescence from the vats caught his eye and aroused his curiosity. He began experimenting with gases or "airs." He bubbled "fixed air" (carbon dioxide) into water and made soda water and also

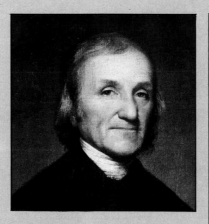

discovered ten new gases including nitrous oxide, ammonia and sulfur dioxide.

A few years later, in 1773, Priestley entered the service of the Earl of Shelburne as resident intellectual and mentor. He continued his scientific work and, in 1774, performed the experiments for which he is famed. On heating red mercuric oxide with a magnifying glass, he collected a colorless gas which made a candle burn vigorously and a mouse live longer than in common air. Inhaling it stimulated him agreeably and he remarked that "this pure air may become a fashionable article in luxury."

Usually so radical in his thinking, Priestley ironically interpreted his discovery according to the traditional phlogiston theory. This held that a substance, burned in air, loses an immaterial principle

called phlogiston which causes the air to become "phlogisticated." Completely phlogisticated air no longer supports combustion or respiration.

Priestley therefore called his gas "dephlogisticated air" — air so pure it contained no phlogiston — and thought of respiration as the "phlogistication of dephlogisticated air." It took the genius of French chemist Antoine Lavoisier to realize that Priestley's "pure air" was pure, not because it lacked some mysterious principle, but because it was a new gas — oxygen.

After leaving the Earl of Shelburne, Priestley lived and worked in Birmingham until, in 1791, his support for the French Revolution caused him to flee. A mob destroyed his house and library to show their disapproval of his views, and when war was declared on France, in 1793, Priestley and his wife left for the United States. They settled in Pennsylvania, where Priestley wrote, entertained such friends as Thomas Jefferson and Benjamin Franklin, and believed in the phlogiston theory till his death in 1804. A great scientist, Priestley is also remembered as a pioneer in education and a defender of individual freedom.

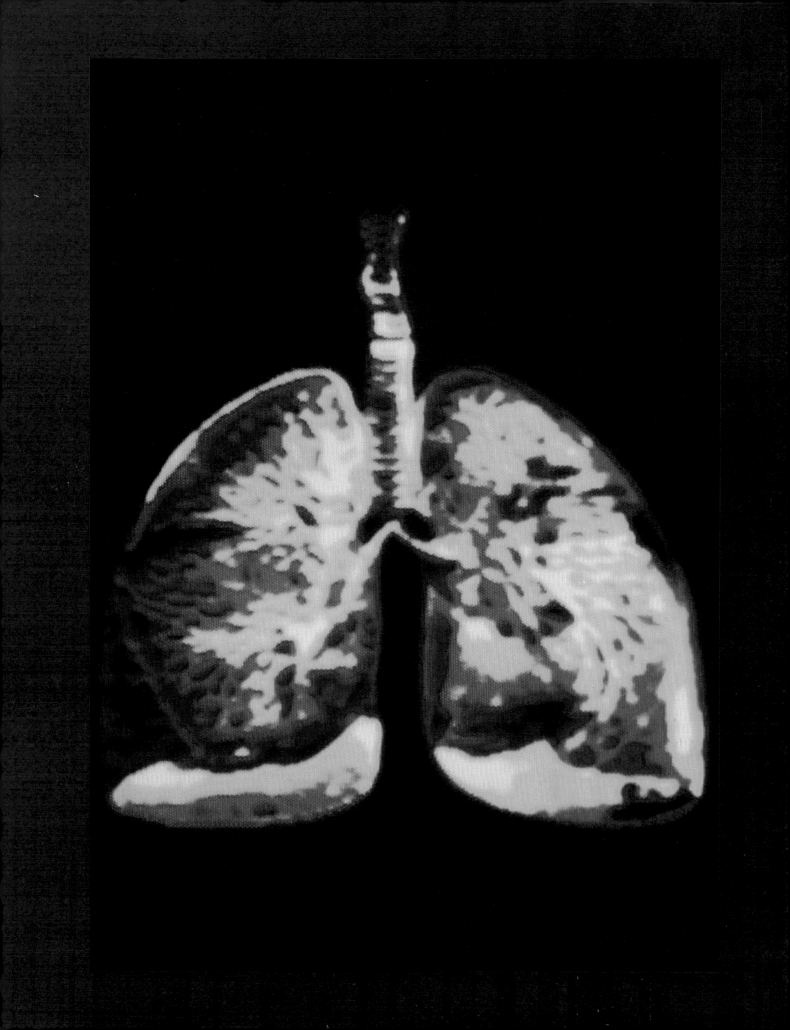

Chapter 2

The Developing System

The success story of mankind, from its beginnings on the plains of Africa a million or more years ago to the incredibly complex and sophisticated lifestyle of today, owes much to intelligence, but this is only part of the secret. Along with all the rest of the mammals and the birds, humans enjoy warm-bloodedness. That is, the temperature of the body is maintained at a high constant level, usually higher than that of the environment. In some tropical areas, the body is maintained at a slightly lower temperature than that of the environment during the day, although in even the hottest deserts, nighttime temperatures fall dramatically. By maintaining a constant temperature, man and other mammals are always ready to react in any circumstance — unlike cold-blooded snakes and lizards which can hardly move in the early morning until the sun's rays have warmed up their cold muscles.

Warm-bloodedness means that all the body's chemical reactions can take place at a fast, predictable rate; this applies to the chemical reactions in the brain and nervous system as much as to the muscles of the limbs. Large quantities of energy are needed to drive these chemical reactions, so mammals require high-quality, reliable food sources as generators of this energy. But until the food which has been eaten is digested and then "burnt" with oxygen — oxidized, as it is termed scientifically — little energy is available to the mammal. Oxidation occurs when oxygen enters the bloodstream and moves to all the cells of the body, where it can take part in the body's chemical industry. The mammalian respiratory system is specifically designed to provide the body with a ready supply of oxygen and, secondarily, to remove gaseous waste products of the oxidative processes, which include carbon dioxide.

But the air we breathe contains a considerable amount of gas for which the body has no use — only one-fifth of it is oxygen. Appropriately, the

By use of a specialized scanning camera, an X ray image can be "sliced" and color coded into its various photographic densities. An X ray of human lungs treated in this way reveals the organ in a dramatic new dimension and provides valuable information about its structure.

A cutaway diagram of the chest, viewed from the front of the body, shows the position of the upper airways, lungs and heart within the thoracic cavity. The diaphragm lies at the base of the lungs.

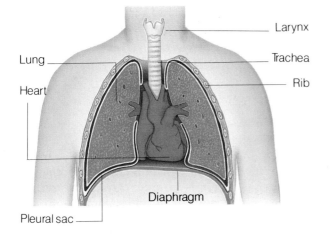

Larynx

Lung

Heart

Trachea

Rib

Diaphragm

Pleural sac

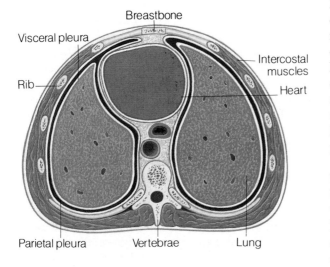

Breastbone

Visceral pleura

Rib

Intercostal muscles

Heart

Parietal pleura

Vertebrae

Lung

A transverse section through the chest shows how the lungs and heart are protected by the bony thoracic cage. This is formed by the breastbone, or sternum, at the front, the ribs on each side and the vertebrae at the back.

respiratory system is extremely efficient at extracting the useful fraction from the air and moving it rapidly to the blood and from there to the mitochondria in every cell of the body. Every human body contains billions of mitochondria, which generate energy-rich compounds from oxidative respiration.

The human respiratory system can be divided into three main sections. The first contains the "pumping machinery," muscles and elastic fibers which pull and push air in and out of the lungs. The second is the system of conducting airways through which air is transported to and from the third region, the lung alveoli. Here, gaseous exchange with the blood occurs.

The Respiratory Pump

Inflation of the lungs — one half of the breathing cycle — is an active, muscular process. Pause a moment to consider the normal human breathing cycle. Starting from nearly empty, or relaxed, lungs, as we breathe in, we can feel our chests expand. But at no time as we fill our lungs do we feel the need for a nonreturn valve somewhere at the back of the throat. This demonstrates that air is held in the lungs under no more than the merest pressure. So how are the lungs inflated?

The answer is that the lungs are similar to two balloons fixed inside a pair of old-fashioned bellows. The balloons are joined at their necks, which project from the bellows as a nozzle. As the handles are forced apart, an area of low pressure is created inside the bellows. One of the basic characteristics of all fluids, and air is a fluid, is that zones of higher and lower pressure are always equaled out. So, as the bellows' handles are opened, the air outside the instrument immediately rushes in through the nozzle to equalize the disparity in pressure, and as a result, the balloons inflate.

The chest cavity is like the body of the bellows, but there are no handles. Instead, there is a tough muscular sheet, the diaphragm, underlying the rib cage, and there is the rib cage itself with muscles between the individual ribs. The lungs are automatically inflated when the diaphragm contracts and pulls downward (so lowering the air pressure in the chest), and the ribs move outward

During the process of photosynthesis, green plants give off oxygen and absorb carbon dioxide. Large-scale destruction of trees, as is taking place in tropical rainforests, potentially affects the atmosphere by increasing the carbon dioxide and decreasing the oxygen content of the air. Increased carbon dioxide in the atmosphere could trap heat that would otherwise escape, possibly causing Earth's temperature to rise.

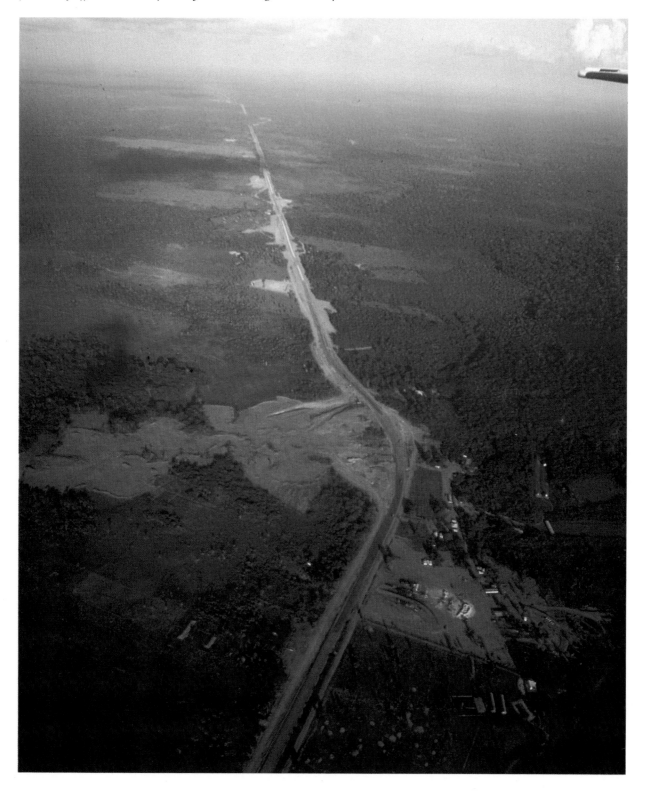

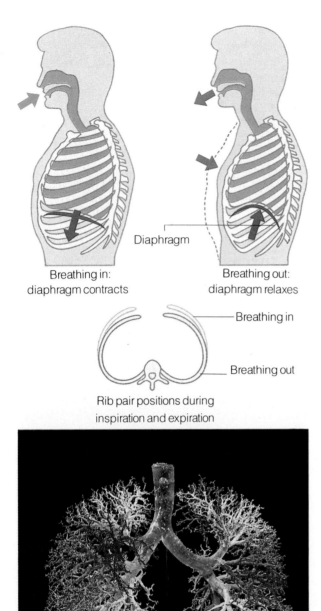

Breathing in:
diaphragm contracts

Diaphragm

Breathing out:
diaphragm relaxes

Breathing in

Breathing out

Rib pair positions during
inspiration and expiration

*The air spaces and associated
airways of the lungs may be used as
a mold for making a cast of these
complex tubes. The resulting 3-D
network reveals the multiple
branching that occurs within the
lungs. In this mold, each lobe of the
lungs is colored differently.*

*When we breathe in, the ribs move
upward and outward and the
diaphragm flattens. On breathing
out, the diaphragm and muscles
associated with the ribs relax, and
the ribs return to their rest position.*

and upward. The lungs themselves play a purely passive role in the inspiratory movement. The changes in volume that they undergo are brought about solely through changes in the capacity of the chest. Continuing the bellows-balloon analogy, the central space of the bellows is represented in the chest by a flattened chamber, the pleural sac, which follows the complex outer contours of the lungs.

Almost two-thirds of the volume of air inspired is due to the pistonlike action of the muscular diaphragm. This structure is an arched sheet of tendinous muscle, attached at the back to the spinal column and at the sides to the lower ribs. In the front it is attached to the tip of the breastbone, or sternum. When the diaphragm contracts, it hardly changes shape — it appears to move downward, and to sit more firmly on the abdomen.

The remaining one-third of the volume of inspired air is the responsibility of the rib cage itself. As we breathe in, the intercostal muscles, which run over, under and between the ribs, pull the ribs upward and outward. To see what happens, stand sideways in front of a mirror: the sternum (breastbone) moves outward as we breathe in. The muscular action of the rib cage and the movement of the ribs themselves is extremely complicated, but try to imagine each rib pair at the relaxed point of the breathing cycle as being like the handle of a bucket lying on its rim. As we breathe in, the ribs move in a similar fashion to the bucket handle moving slightly upward from its resting position.

Breathing out, or expiration, is a much simpler process than breathing in. At the end of the so-called inspirational phase, the intercostal muscles and the diaphragm muscles relax, and the chest cavity elastically recoils to its previous volume. In addition, the elasticity of the lungs themselves helps dispel air from them.

If we wish to breathe out somewhat faster than normal — if, for example, we are running or otherwise active — expiration will be assisted by a contraction of the abdominal and some intercostal muscles, which will forcefully push the diaphragm upward into the thorax. During heavy breathing, one or two other events occur to make the passage of air more free. The nostrils flare slightly, and the opening between the vocal cords (the glottis) enlarges. Certain muscles at the front of the neck

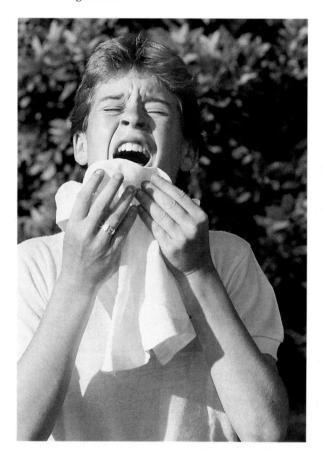

A sneeze is a reflex action designed to clear irritation from the upper respiratory tract. Air may be expelled at up to 103 miles per hour and carry 100,000 droplets of mucus and microorganisms.

may also assist by pulling the top rib of the chest upward. Since this is attached via tendons to the sternum, the breastbone is also lifted upward and slightly outward.

Airways and Alveoli

The air that is sucked into the lungs during inspiration passes along a series of tubes which take it from the outside to the substance of the lungs. The upper part of this tube system, the respiratory airways, consists of the mouth and nose cavities and the single trachea, or windpipe. Below, in the chest, it divides into two bronchi, one of which passes into each lung. Each bronchus then branches, or subdivides, about eighteen times to produce a treelike, spreading network of finer and finer air tunnels.

The ultimate subdivisions of the airways of each lung are extremely thin tubes, the bronchioles. At the ends of these bronchioles are the areas where gas exchange with the blood occurs — the working zone of the lung. Known as alveoli, these areas consist of minute rounded air spaces surrounded by capillaries of the blood system of the lungs.

The normal breathing cycle operated by these three parts of the system sometimes alters, however. Familiar actions such as coughing, yawning, hiccuping and sneezing are all simply modifications of the system — each with its own purpose.

Coughing, Sneezing and Yawning

A cough differs only from normal expiration in its ferocity. The fast-moving wave of air, greatly accelerated by a huge contraction of the abdominal muscles, passes like a whirlwind up the airway and through a nearly closed glottis, carrying lumps of mucus in its wake. Prolonged coughing may be needed if the amount of gluey mucus to be moved is large. When we clear our throats, we bring about the same effect, the only difference being that throat-clearing can be carefully and accurately controlled.

Another variant of normal breathing, sneezing, is, like coughing, a means of clearing small irritations from the upper respiratory tract. Any irritation of the mucous membrane lining of the upper tract will induce sneezing; hayfever sufferers

know all too well the effect of fine dust and grass pollen on the sneezing response. There are well-publicized cases of people who cannot stop sneezing, but such are rare; usually sneezing ceases when the irritation has been appeased.

The hiccup, a little-understood phenomenon of no great significance, is an involuntary inspiration, led by a rapid contraction of the diaphragm. A blow to the solar plexus is sufficient to induce an attack of hiccups, so it would appear that the autonomic nervous system, whose nerves emanate from this site, is somehow involved. There are many folk-cures for hiccups, most of which seem to rely upon a short, sharp shock. Babies sometimes suffer from hiccups before they are born, and this can readily be felt by their mothers.

Yawning, an even more common occurrence, is the body's response to a buildup of carbon dioxide in the lungs. The levels of oxygen and carbon dioxide in the blood are constantly monitored by,

29

A yawn is a long, involuntary inhalation with wide-open mouth, usually in response to a high carbon dioxide level in the lungs. In 1888, a fifteen-year-old American girl was recorded as yawning for five weeks.

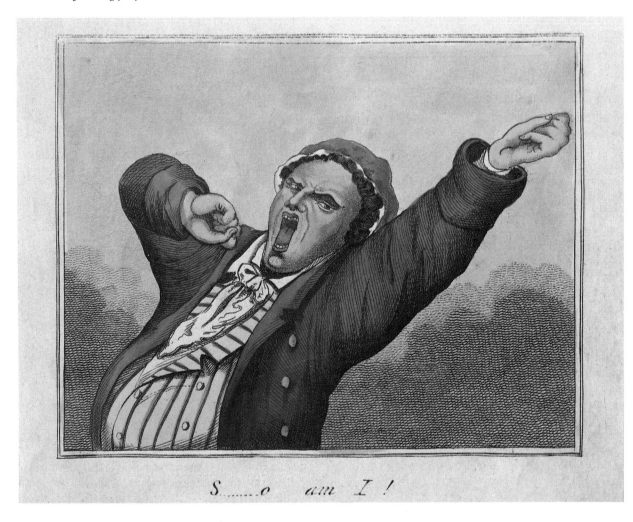

S____o am I !

among other organs, special "respiratory centers" situated at the base of the brain. When we are tired, and often when sitting still, our breathing becomes shallower and less gas is cleared from the lungs; also, more carbon dioxide is produced at these times. All of a sudden, the respiratory center calls upon us to flush out our lungs, and it is a call that is hard to disobey. Yawning is not under the sole control of the respiratory center, however, for it is a socially infectious habit, although the reason why we should feel the urge to yawn when we see someone else yawning is not known.

Respiration in other Vertebrates

This brief review of the basic anatomy and functioning of the respiratory system applies to man and other mammals. But we and our mammalian relatives are the product of millions of years of evolution, during which a basic vertebrate plan has been modified and adapted. In order to understand more fully our own seemingly complicated system of respiration, it is helpful to understand the evolutionary changes that have occurred.

The story begins some 300 to 400 million years ago, when ancient relatives of the sharks abounded in the oceans. (Bony fishes, the forerunners of modern fishes such as cod and sole, evolved a little later.) Vertebrates that live in water possess special structures, gills, for extracting oxygen from the water. An examination of a present-day shark will show that there are five to seven slits on each side of the head and a small hole in front of the most forward slit; these are the gill slits. The shark obtains oxygen by taking in water through its mouth and expelling it through the gill slits, each of which contains many fingerlike flaps of tissue, richly supplied with blood. The single ventricle, or lower chamber of the heart, which lies more or less in front of the shark's front fins, pumps blood into the gill slits, and here oxygen diffuses from the water through the thin walls of the tiny "fingers" and into the blood.

The blood vessels now pass backward along the roof of the mouth as the main artery, with small arteries branching off to deliver oxygenated blood to all parts of the body. Once the blood has given up its oxygen in the tissues and collected its load of waste carbon dioxide, it returns to the single auricle, or upper chamber of the heart, via a series of thin-walled veins. From the auricle it passes into the ventricle to be pumped once more to the gills. The points to note are that there are five to seven gill slits, each with its own blood supply, and that the blood's circulation is similar to a child's circular model railroad track, in which the toy train travels relentlessly round and round.

The situation in bony fishes is somewhat similar, except that the gill slits are covered by a bony flap, or operculum, as can be seen when a trout is being prepared for cooking. There are five gill slits, or spaces, between the pink, spongy gill filaments, as the fingerlike projections are correctly called. As in the shark, blood is pumped forward from a simple two-chambered heart through the gills, where oxygen is obtained, and is then collected by a series of small vessels which join to produce the dorsal aorta, just as in the shark.

There is one group of bony fishes, however, which deserves special mention. These are the lungfishes, so called because they have a simple lung — a pocket built out from the gut — to allow them to breathe air when their muddy pools become stagnant and dry up.

Modern lungfishes — there are just six species, one each in South America and Australia and four in Africa — have a reduced number of gills, but they have a blood system similar to that of other fishes. Just at the start of the dorsal aorta, a side branch, the pulmonary artery, runs to the lung. This structure bears little resemblance to the mammalian lung,

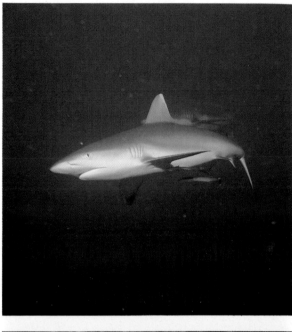

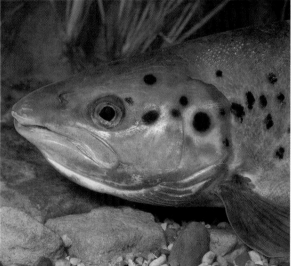

In bony fishes the gill openings are covered by a flap, the operculum, so making only one effective opening on each side of the head. Water, containing oxygen, is pumped continuously over the gills by muscles around the mouth and opercular cavity. Fishes use up to 80 percent of the oxygen contained in water.

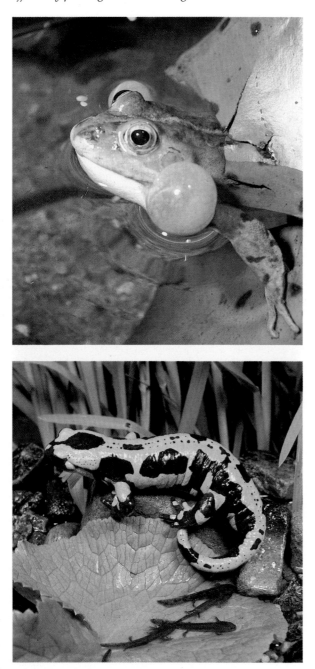

Amphibians, such as this salamander, obtain much of their oxygen directly through the body. The skin is extremely thin and, provided it stays moist, oxygen can diffuse across it into the lungs.

being little more than a simple, thin-walled bag. The pulmonary artery divides in the lung to form a filigree of small vessels, which join in the lower aspect of the lung to form a pulmonary vein. The auricle is partly divided, so oxygen-rich blood from the lung does not mix too much with depleted blood, and the ventricle is almost completely divided by a series of muscular ridges.

In evolutionary terms, lungfishes show that, even among some of the earliest vertebrate animals, an air-breathing life was physiologically possible. In fact, the first amphibians, ancient relatives of modern salamanders, frogs and toads, made their appearance some 350 million years ago in the late Devonian and early Carboniferous eras.

Amphibians were the first vertebrate animals to exploit some of the advantages of life on dry land, although their conversion to a terrestrial life was not a complete one. Even modern amphibians must, for instance, retain a moist skin in order to obtain sufficient oxygen from the air and must return to water to breed. Fossils show that the early amphibians were heavy, lumbering animals which would have been able to move about only slowly and with difficulty. But amphibians do possess recognizable lungs, which stretch into the chest from the back of the mouth.

The amphibians have no diaphragm (and therefore no enclosed thoracic cavity) nor inter-costal muscle system, so ventilation is poor. It is effected by "gulping" — a motion easily seen in frogs — in which air is pulled into the mouth via the nostrils and sent down to the lungs. By repeatedly raising and lowering the floor of the mouth, while the nostrils and mouth are kept tightly shut, the lungs are emptied and filled again with the same air. It is thought that this somewhat odd practice results in maximum gaseous interchange with minimum water loss, for every time air is expelled from the body, precious water is lost. This method of using the floor of the mouth to take in air is clearly derived from the movements of the floor of the mouth in fish, by which water is forced over the gills.

All larval amphibians, and some (such as the common mud puppy) in adult form, have external gills. In them the blood-circulatory system is recognizably similar to the basic gill-slit system

In the cardiac-related blood systems of the amphibian, reptile and mammal (below) the single lines represent blood vessels derived through evolution from former gill blood vessels or other such vessels.

Cardiac-related vertebrate blood systems

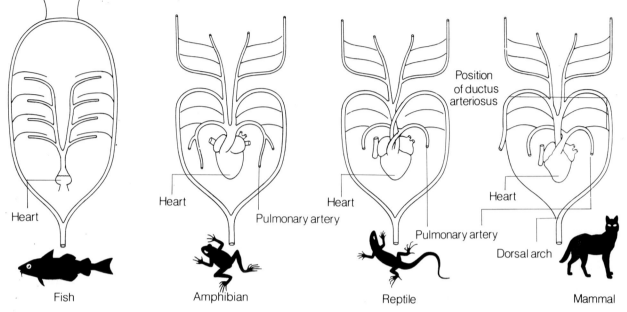

Heart

Fish

Heart
Pulmonary artery

Amphibian

Heart
Pulmonary artery

Reptile

Position of ductus arteriosus

Heart
Dorsal arch

Mammal

found in fish. In the more terrestrial amphibians, such as frogs and toads, the start of a circulation bearing similarities to that of the higher mammals is evident. Mud puppies, axolotls and several other amphibians have three pairs of gills and five gill slits. The ventral aorta supplies them with venous blood, and the dorsal aorta carries away oxygen-enriched blood. The pulmonary artery still goes to the tiny lungs, but little oxygen, if any, is picked up by the returning pulmonary vein.

Frogs and toads have neither gills nor gill slits and pump oxygen-poor blood to the lungs. This returns to a divided left auricle, from where it is pumped around the body via the dorsal aorta. Notwithstanding the apparent sophistication of the frog's circulatory system, much gaseous exchange between the air and the animal's blood circulation takes place through the skin, and particularly through the skin of the mouth.

The earliest amphibians gave rise, some 330 million years ago, to a group of creatures that were able to lay their eggs on dry land. From this early beginning sprang the reptiles and birds, whose modern representatives lay eggs, and mammals, which mostly do not. Effectively no direct diffusion of oxygen takes place across the skin surface of reptiles, birds and mammals, even in the water-dwelling species such as whales and dolphins. Frequently the skin is armor plated with scales for protection, or covered with feathers or hair.

Respiration in these animals depends solely upon a pair of lungs. In reptiles, as in birds, it is the anterior, or forward, part of the lung that acts as the respiratory organ. The rear part is often devoid of any blood vessels and serves as an air reservoir into, and out of, which air can be moved. This system is also employed in amphibians.

The reptilian heart has four chambers, but they are not fully separated. Whereas a mammal has a single aorta, reptiles have two aortas, which are supplied with mostly arterial, oxygen-rich blood. The pulmonary artery receives mostly venous, oxygen-poor blood, but there is some mixing in all vessels. In only one group of reptiles, the crocodiles, is the division of the heart into four separate chambers almost complete. And in this group of reptiles also, a kind of diaphragm occurs; this is not directly analogous to the mammalian diaphragm, but it serves a somewhat similar purpose.

It is currently thought that some of the dinosaurs were warm-blooded, active creatures which could hunt at night and in the winter. Many zoologists regard birds as the closest living relatives of the

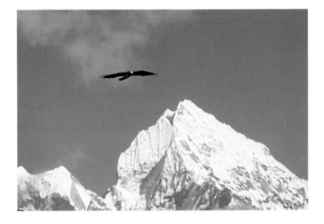

dinosaurs, and they possess warm blood and a constant body temperature, as well as a four-chambered, perfectly divided heart.

In birds, the circulatory system is typified by a single aorta, or systemic arch; it sweeps around to the right, while in mammals it loops to the left, but otherwise the two are similar. The bird's pulmonary circulation operates at low pressure, and the lung capillary system is often said to constitute the most efficient of vertebrate respiratory systems. Certainly, birds are able to fly at heights in excess of 33,000 feet, where oxygen levels are extremely low and at which altitude mammals die.

A bird's lung is small and compact, slightly resembling an automobile radiator through which water is passed. Gaseous exchange takes place in a network of tiny chambers, each less than one seventy-fifth of an inch in length. Air is passed through this network and then stored in a complicated series of air sacs, which lie in the chest and abdomen and even extend into the thighs and the centers of bones. These air sacs may serve the secondary function of insulating the deeper tissues from low temperatures such as are experienced when flying at great heights. They also reduce the weight of the body — an important consideration in a flying vertebrate. When the bird breathes in, it is, however, thought that the air bypasses the lungs and immediately enters the posterior air sacs, from where it traverses the lung and then enters the more anterior air sacs (placed farther forward).

This brief review has shown something of the fate of the basic components of the vertebrate respiratory and circulatory systems. Mammalian respiration is a refined version of those systems of the lower orders of vertebrates, and it utilizes only three of the original six sets of respiratory arteries. In fishes, the sixth set, like all the others, joins the ventral aorta with the dorsal aorta. In mammals, the sixth set forms the pulmonary arteries, leading deoxygenated blood to the lungs. But before birth, when the lungs are not functional, the pulmonary arteries revert to their ancient role, and certain anatomical changes must occur when the newborn mammal makes its entry into the air-breathing world and draws its first breath.

The Developing Lungs

The development of the human lungs in an embryo within the womb begins when the head-to-rump length is a mere one-tenth of an inch. At that stage, an outpocketing occurs on the ventral side of the front region of the gut. From this will grow the lungs, which are, developmentally, an extension of the alimentary tract. The growing gut extension then divides into two, giving the rudiments of the main right and left bronchi. It splits again into three on the right side and two on the left, beginning the process of successive subdivisions of the bronchial tree. Throughout embryonic and fetal development, the lungs are filled with fluid.

The human fetus requires a good blood system to transport nutrients from the placenta around its rapidly growing body and to shift metabolic wastes back to the placenta, so a blood system develops early on in fetal life. As the fetus does not breathe air, the lungs are nonfunctional at this stage. For the first four and a half months of human pregnancy, there is a hole in the wall between the right and left atria of the heart (the chambers equivalent to the auricles in other vertebrates), and blood flows from the right to the left atrium — a valvelike flap of tissue prevents the movement of blood in the opposite direction. This keeps most of the blood out of the right ventricle and so out of the pulmonary arteries and embryonic lungs.

During the second half of pregnancy, this hole starts to close up and should have closed completely by birth. The effect of this is to ensure that the right ventricle receives blood and sends it, via the pulmonary artery, to the lungs. Before birth, however, the pulmonary artery retains a functional

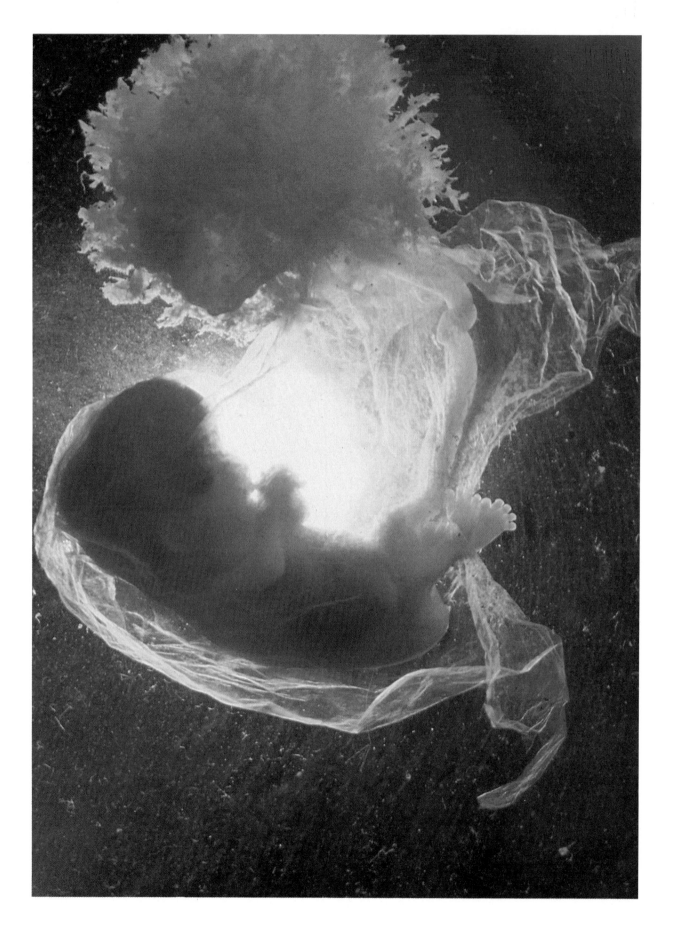

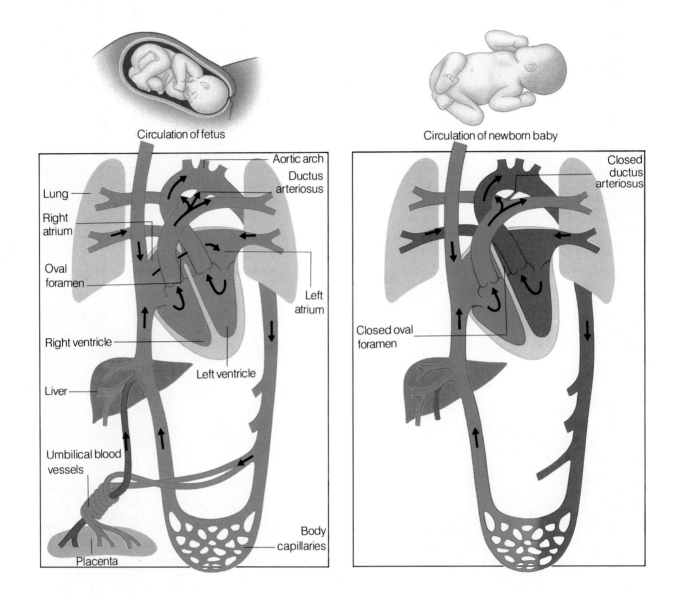

Circulation of fetus

Circulation of newborn baby

Aortic arch

Ductus arteriosus

Lung

Right atrium

Oval foramen

Left atrium

Right ventricle

Left ventricle

Liver

Umbilical blood vessels

Placenta

Body capillaries

Closed ductus arteriosus

Closed oval foramen

While a baby is in the womb, oxygenated blood from the placenta flows to the right side of the heart. Most then flows to the left side of the heart through the oval foramen, "the hole in the heart," and is pumped around the body. At birth the circulation must change. The hole in the heart should already be closing, and the passage which bypasses the lung circulation is beginning to close off. Once the lungs are inflated with air by the first breath, blood is forced from the right side of the heart into the lung circulation, and the full respiratory system starts to operate.

connection with the dorsal aorta, so resembling the situation found in the respiratory systems of fishes and larval amphibians.

The connection is known by its Latin name of ductus arteriosus. It is about half an inch long in the newborn and about a quarter of an inch in diameter. The effect of birth on the fetal diaphragm induces the first intake of air, and the lungs ventilate. Within a few minutes, the ductus arteriosus begins to contract and should close completely between the fourth and the tenth day after birth. Similarly, the hole between the two atria should also have closed by the tenth day, but a small slit — all that is left of the valvelike structure — sometimes persists for longer. It is not known for certain what causes the ductus arteriosus to close, but it is thought that contraction of its own smooth musculature has a great deal to do with it, and particular hormones, prostaglandins, have also been identified as playing a role. Gradually the ductus becomes fibrous, and it persists throughout life as a band joining the pulmonary artery to the dorsal aorta.

The First Breath

The fetal lung is not in a collapsed state. It is actually inflated, with a special liquid secreted by the alveolar cells, to about 40 percent of its total capacity. Physiologists now think that the function of this fluid, which contains a natural "detergent," surfactant, is to help reduce the large surface tension forces in the alveoli that have to be overcome in the first breath. The fetus is known to make small breathing movements in the few weeks before birth, and one effect of this is to squeeze excess fluid out of the lungs. Once the first breath is taken, surfactant helps to keep the alveoli open, and excess lung fluid is absorbed into the bloodstream. However, it takes several days before uniform ventilation is achieved.

Before birth, the human baby has to rely on its mother's respiratory system for its oxygen supply. Gaseous exchange between mother and baby takes place in the placenta, but, since the barrier across which oxygen has to pass is many times thicker than the alveolar barrier in the lung, the exchange is not very efficient. However, the oxygenated blood leaves the placental capillary bed by means of the umbilical vein. Most of this blood enters the left atrium via the hole in the wall between left and right atria and then flows from the left ventricle to the rest of the body.

What this arrangement ensures is that the most highly oxygenated blood — even so, it is poor by adult standards — goes to the brain and to the heart itself, for these are key organs in the development of the baby. Following birth and the expulsion of the placenta, with the severing of all interchange between mother and baby, the umbilical vein quickly starts to collapse. At between two and five days after birth, it has dwindled to a fibrous cord seen, in adults, as a ligament around the liver.

Birth, then, brings about this amazing series of respiratory changes. Within a week of birth, the baby has changed entirely from being an appendage of its mother to being a free-living creature and is fully embarked on the five hundred million to one billion breaths it might expect to take in a seventy-year lifespan.

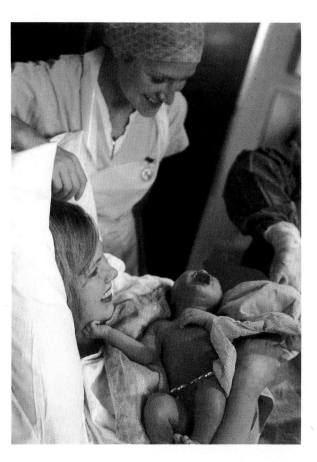

A baby's first breath, often combined with a loud cry, is a dramatic thrilling sign that all is well. Nowadays most doctors allow a few moments for breathing to become established before cutting the umbilical cord and severing the oxygen supply from the placenta. Most babies breathe at a rate of about thirty-three to forty breaths a minute, much faster than the adult rate of about fourteen breaths a minute.

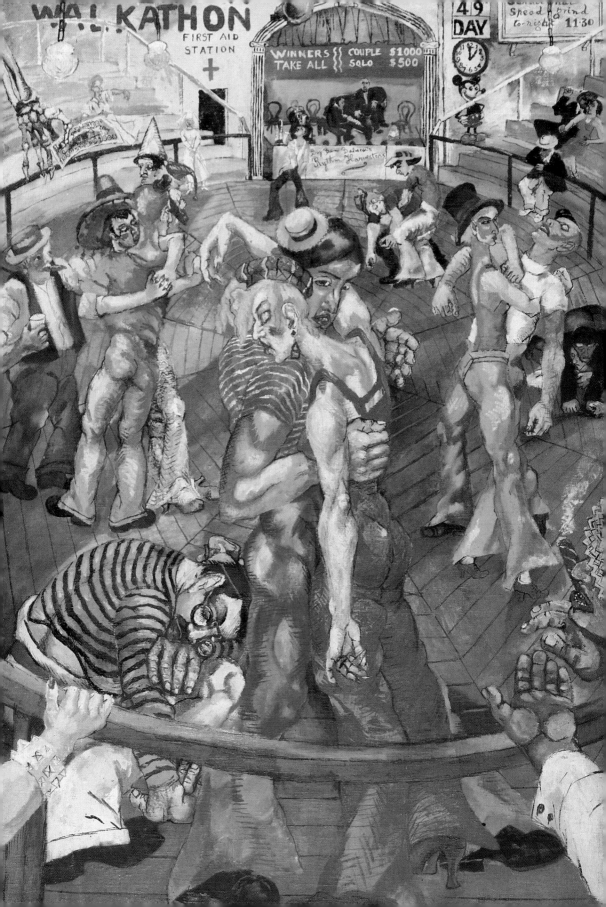

Chapter 3

The Mechanics of Breathing

The air we breathe is the first essential for life. Without the oxygen it contains, the cells of the human body cannot function, cannot exploit the energy resources available to them and death ensues. The true nature of oxygen as the life-supporting gas was realized by the great French scientist Antoine Lavoisier in 1775, and this understanding of the nature of respiration was one of the major scientific contributions of the eighteenth century.

The lungs are the organs of respiration; they carry oxygen from the air to the blood and pass carbon dioxide from the blood to be expelled with the outgoing breath. Two membranes separate the lungs from the chest wall. The inner pleural membrane is attached to the lungs themselves, the outer to the inner margins of the ribs. When the lungs and rib cage move relative to one another during breathing, the only surfaces that actually move past one another are the inner linings of the two pleural membranes. The gap between them is filled with a thin layer of fluid which acts as a lubricant, enabling lungs and rib cage to slide easily without friction.

Air reaches the lungs via the interconnecting series of tubes and passageways that make up the conducting airways. Air usually enters the body through the nose, but during periods of exertion, when the demand for air is high, it also enters through the mouth. For a number of reasons it is better for the nostrils to be the point of entry, for their rims and the small cavity just behind them are both covered with small hairs which filter dust and other particles from the air. The nasal cavity itself is lined with a mucous membrane, and a thick, sticky sheet of mucus is driven forward toward the nostrils by the hairs. Particles which have slipped through the net of hairs are entangled in the mucus, and only clean air passes onward to the lungs. The mucous membrane also serves to humidify the air and to correct its temperature.

The activity of the human body is fueled by oxygen. Without it, energy resources cannot be unlocked and the body cannot function. But, given air to breathe, human beings are capable of remarkable physical endurance. Participants in the gruelling dance marathons of the thirties, here depicted by Philip Evergood, would dance around the clock for days on end, in the hope of winning a prize, until they collapsed from sheer physical exhaustion.

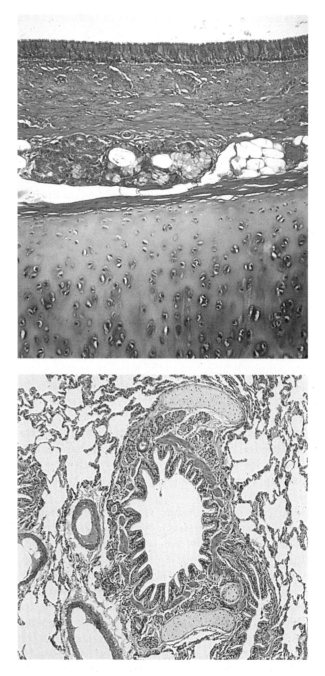

After it leaves the nasal cavity, the air passes backward and downward through the larynx. A complicated structure of thin bone, cartilage and muscles, the larynx is the site of speech. The air passes between the relaxed vocal cords through what is known as the glottis. Compare the rate at which air normally passes through the glottis with the much slower rate when we contract the vocal cords and try to speak on an indrawn breath. One of the difficulties with human speech is that it severely restricts the flow rate of air into the lungs. Inexperienced lecturers sometimes report symptoms of dizziness and being short of breath if they speak too fast and do not allow themselves time to breathe properly.

Immediately beneath the larynx is the windpipe, or trachea. This is almost four and a half inches long and between three-quarters of an inch and an inch in diameter. It is slightly larger in men than in women. The main characteristic of the vertebrate trachea — clearly seen by anybody who has prepared a chicken or rabbit for cooking — is that it is reinforced by bands of stiff gristle or cartilage. These do not completely surround the tube, since a small gap is left at the back of the windpipe, but this is filled with a band of strong fibers that keep this major air passage open at all times.

The Bronchial Tree

At its bottom end, the trachea forks into two short, stubby tubes known as the bronchi. Each bronchus is about one inch in length, and each is stiffened with cartilage hoops. The right bronchus branches again almost immediately because the right lung is divided into three parts, or lobes, while the left lung is divided into only two. This branching occurs again and again until a "tree" is created. Gradually the stiffening cartilage hoops become more sparse until they are little more than randomly scattered plates of the thinnest material. Finally, at the level of the smallest "twigs" of the tree, this system of airways comes to an end.

These most slender vessels in the bronchial tree are known as bronchioles, and they are typified by an absence of cartilaginous rings. They are less than one twenty-fifth of an inch in diameter and have muscle fibers that run around them like numerous rubber bands.

The surfaces of the larynx, trachea and bronchi (A) are ringed with C-shaped hoops of cartilage which strengthen the airways and prevent them collapsing in the event of significant pressure change. A section of the trachea (B) shows the layers of muscle and cartilage within the airway wall. The bronchi bear smaller cartilage hoops than the trachea, and the tiny bronchioles lack cartilage.

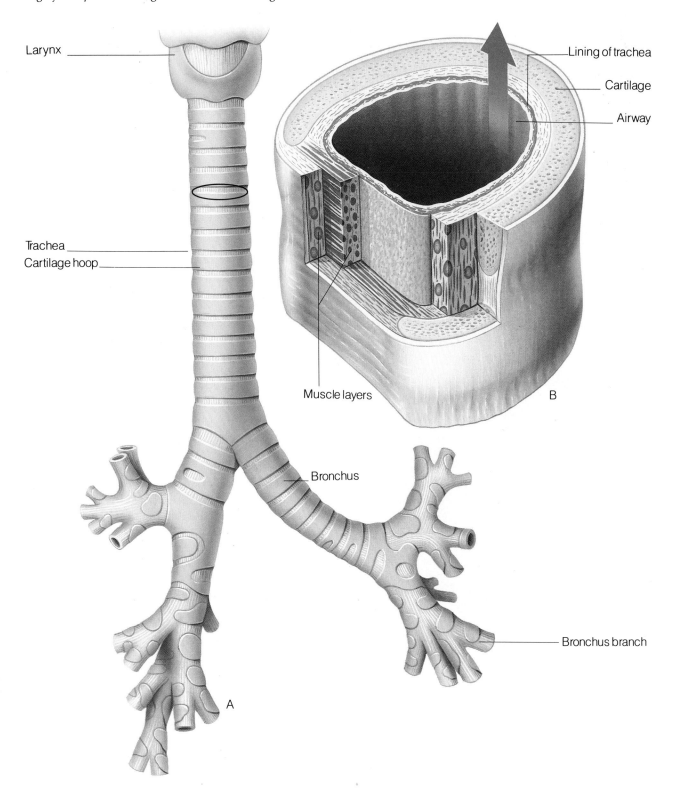

Larynx

Lining of trachea

Cartilage

Airway

Trachea

Cartilage hoop

Muscle layers

B

Bronchus

A

Bronchus branch

Hairlike cilia, here magnified about 7,000 times, project from the airways and propel mucus, secreted by the lining, into the throat and away from the lungs. The mucus traps any particles in the airways.

The cellular lining of the airways normally carry cilia (A), which beat with a wavelike motion (C) to move mucus. Prolonged cigarette smoking damages the lining and eventually destroys the cilia (B).

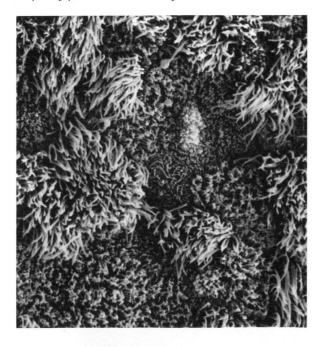

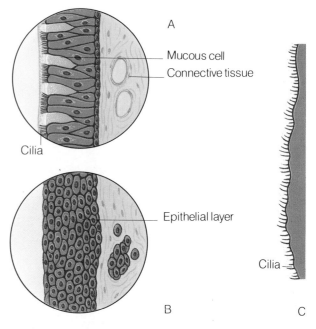

A

Mucous cell
Connective tissue

Cilia

Epithelial layer

Cilia

B

C

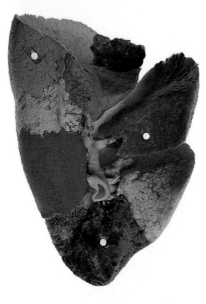

A human right lung injected with colored dyes shows the zones of lung tissue supplied by different branches of the airway system. The right lung is larger than the left, which must share chest space with the heart.

All the pipes and passages in the respiratory airways are lined with a mucous membrane and bear countless millions of tiny hairlike projections, known as cilia. These beat upward, so driving the mucus toward the throat and away from the lungs. As in the nose, the function of the mucus secreted from glands is to entrap tiny particles that might damage the tissues of the lungs. The mucous membrane, however, provides a potential breeding ground for bacteria; various of these organisms are specialized for life in the trachea (giving rise to tracheitis), and in the bronchi and bronchioles (bronchitis). When under attack from these organisms, the glands in the membrane respond by producing increased quantities of thick mucus. The action of the cilia can only move this slowly, but coughing can induce a more rapid movement of the mucus layer. One of the many harmful effects of smoking is that the action of the cilia is damaged and mucus becomes thicker and more liable to be retained. The characteristic smoker's cough is an attempt to expel the mucus.

The bronchioles, the ultimate branches of the bronchial tree, connect to the alveoli, the lungs' vast surface area for gas exchange — between sixty and one hundred and twenty square yards in all. It is possible to pack this immense surface area into

Antoine-Laurent Lavoisier

Father of Modern Chemistry

"Of all the phenomena of the animal Economy, none is more striking, none more worthy of the attention of philosophers than those which accompany respiration." So wrote Antoine Lavoisier, the brilliant scientist who gave oxygen its name and laid the foundations of modern chemistry.

Born in Paris in 1743, Lavoisier was educated at the Collège Mazarin, where he studied mathematics, astronomy, chemistry and botany, as well as his principle subject, law. On graduation he bought his way into the Ferme Générale — a privately owned tax-gathering monopoly controlled by the monarchy. A public-spirited man, he worked to improve social and economic conditions, instigated insurance schemes and was instrumental in the introduction of metric weights and measures. He also experimented with scientific agriculture and improved the manufacture of gunpowder.

Lavoisier was married, in 1771, to fourteen-year-old Marie-Anne Paulze with whom he had an harmonious but childless marriage. His wife translated English scientific books and papers for him and also mastered engraving and draftsmanship to illustrate his books. She became the greatest advocate of the new chemistry her husband was developing.

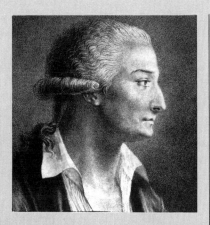

Lavoisier was convinced that chemistry needed accurate quantitative measurements and a clear language with which to describe chemical events. He focused his attention on combustion — one of the chief mysteries of eighteenth century chemistry. By heating substances such as sulfur and phosphorus in controlled conditions, he showed that the resulting changes in weight — of solid or gas — was vital to the understanding of combustion.

After Joseph Priestley visited Lavoisier in 1774 and told him of his "dephlogisticated air," Lavoisier worked on Priestley's mercuric oxide experiment — but reversed it. Under controlled conditions he showed that "dephlogisticated air" was a new element which he named "oxigine." Derived from a Greek word meaning "the begetter of acids," this name summarized Lavoisier's belief (found to be erroneous some fifty years later) that all acids contain this gas, this "eminently respirable air."

The flaws in the phlogiston theory exposed, Lavoisier turned his attention to respiration. In a series of experiments, begun in 1776, he started to unravel the true story of the interchange of gases in the lungs. He showed that it was oxygen that was used by the lungs, while the bulk of air — known after 1790 as nitrogen — played no part in respiration.

Having demonstrated that carbon dioxide and water were present in expired air, Lavoisier drew a firm analogy between respiration and combustion. He suggested that the body's carbon and hydrogen were oxidized by oxygen, with carbon dioxide as a waste product. He also suggested that, since mercury and lead form red powders with oxygen, it was the absorption of oxygen that gave arterial blood its bright red color.

Lavoisier's life was cut short while he was at the peak of his scientific powers. The hated tax-collectors were major targets of the French Revolutionaries and, in 1794, Lavoisier was executed for "plotting against the people of France." Friend and coworker Laplace said of him: "It took only a moment to sever that head and perhaps a century will not be sufficient to produce another like it."

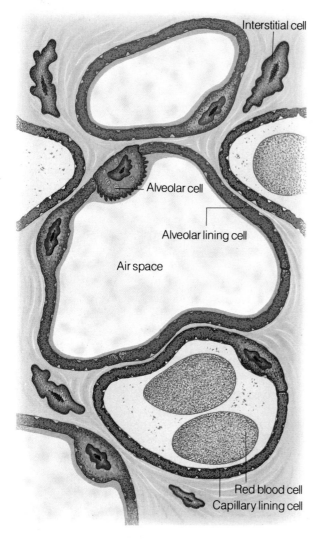

The close proximity of alveolar air spaces and capillary blood, seen in this section through the alveoli and pulmonary capillaries, enables exchange of oxygen and carbon dioxide to take place. Oxygen passes across the alveolar wall and into the blood to be taken up by hemoglobin in the red blood cells. Carbon dioxide, which has been carried from the cells as waste matter, passes into the alveoli to be exhaled.

Interstitial cell

Alveolar cell

Alveolar lining cell

Air space

Red blood cell
Capillary lining cell

the chest cavity because it is subdivided into so many minute sections — there are seven hundred and fifty million or so alveoli in a pair of lungs.

Alveoli resemble bunches of grapes hanging from the bronchioles but are more accurately compared to bunches of tiny balloons, with the thin fabric of the alveolar wall forming the interface for gas exchange with the pulmonary capillaries. The wall of an alveolus is extremely thin, only 0.5 microns across. Such dimensions are hard to imagine, but if a one-centimeter piece of sausage were cut into slices 0.5 microns thick, no fewer than two thousand slices would result.

The Exchange of Gases

Surrounding the alveoli are the pulmonary capillaries, a dense network of narrow, thin-walled blood vessels, the diameter of which is hardly greater than that of a red blood cell. The capillary walls, like those of the alveoli, are thin enough for gas transfer to take place across them with ease; oxygen is picked up and carbon dioxide eliminated. Oxygen is carried to the cells — and carbon dioxide taken away — by the blood. Most of the oxygen is carried in the red blood corpuscles in combination with hemoglobin, the substance that gives blood its red color, although some oxygen is carried dissolved in the blood. All the cells of the body need oxygen to fuel their internal functioning — their metabolism — and, in turn, they produce carbon dioxide as a waste product. Other waste products, including water, are produced by the cells, but these are excreted by other organs, mainly the kidneys.

Breathing out is largely a passive process, the elastic recoil of the lungs causes them to return to their original shape, thus pushing air out. During a forced expiration, all the accessory muscles work to expel air from the lungs.

A term used in definitions of breathing activity is compliance, which describes the responsiveness of the lung volume to muscular or other efforts to change it. Lungs which expand and contract easily have high compliance. "Stiffer" lungs, which change less in volume with similar effort, have low compliance. One important factor affecting the compliance of the lungs is the surface tension of the fluid lining the alveoli. Since 1929, it has been

Blood flows into the lung capillaries (A) for oxygenation and then back to the heart to be pumped around the rest of the body. Each alveolus (B) is surrounded by blood capillaries, and it is here that gas exchange takes place; the walls of both capillaries and alveolus are so thin that gases diffuse across them. As blood passes through the capillaries it collects oxygen and gives up carbon dioxide, which is then exhaled.

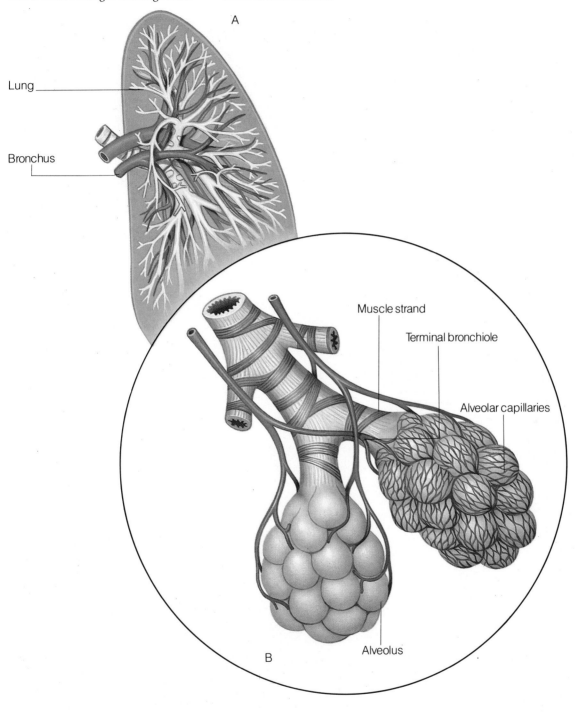

A

Lung

Bronchus

Muscle strand

Terminal bronchiole

Alveolar capillaries

Alveolus

B

An exhalation of breath creates air turbulence made visible by a particular photographic technique. In schlieren photography, the camera records the deflection of light rays caused by changes in the air.

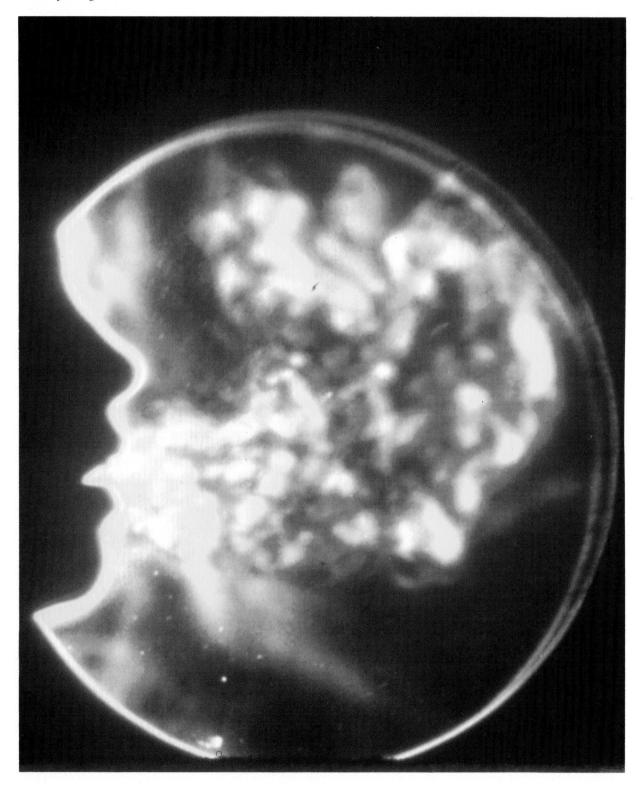

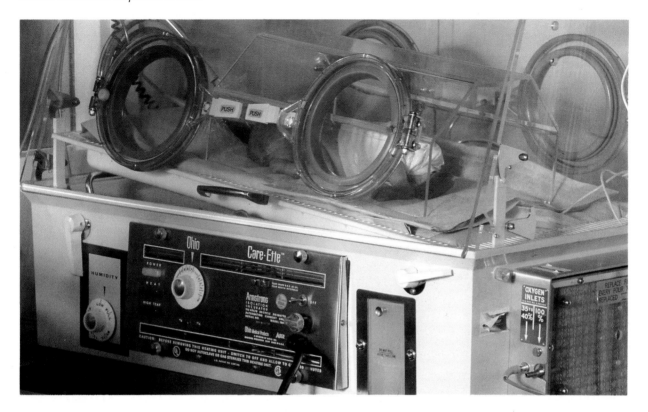

known that isolated lungs (lungs removed from the body) were easier to blow up if they contained fluid as well as air, so demonstrating that fluid-containing lungs are more compliant. Only recently, however, has the nature of this fluid, surfactant, been understood.

The Role of Surfactant

Surfactant is a detergentlike substance that lines all the alveoli and is a complicated mixture of protein and lipid (fat); its main component is dipalmitoyl lecithin. When, during expiration, the alveoli become small, the surfactant molecules are pushed closer together, so reducing the surface tension and preventing the alveoli from collapsing. When the alveoli are expanded, the surfactant is more spread out, but the force tending to cause the alveoli to collapse is much smaller. The balloon analogy is again appropriate. Considerable effort is needed to blow up the first part of a balloon but, once it is partially expanded, inflation becomes easier. In the same way, the forces that tend to collapse the alveoli are at their greatest at the end of

expiration, when the alveoli are at their smallest.

Premature babies, those born weeks before the physiologically "correct" time, may suffer severe problems with lung function, which are generally described by the term respiratory distress syndrome, or RDS. One cause of these problems is a lack of surfactant, which the lungs of the premature baby are not sufficiently developed to produce. Without the correct amount of this substance to lower the surface tension of its lungs, it is difficult for the baby adequately to inflate its fluid-filled lungs with air. Consequently, lung function is poor and the lining layers of the airways rapidly suffer damage. Normally the transition from the fluid-filled lungs of the fetus to air-filled lungs is achieved at the time of the first breath. Premature babies suffering from respiratory distress syndrome must receive immediate intensive care and be helped to breathe.

RDS affects some forty to fifty thousand babies a year in the United States, but developments in treatment over the last twenty years have dramatically reduced the mortality rate.

Layer by layer, the structure of the human respiratory system is revealed in this series of images.

A shows the left side of the upper skeleton of an adult. Surface tissues have been removed to reveal bone details and muscles. The left arm and side wall of the chest cavity are also removed, exposing the left lung and part of the diaphragm.

B shows the central (medial) surface of the left lung, revealing the airways and blood vessels which pass into it.

In C, the upper part of the respiratory tract has been vertically (sagittally) cut to reveal details of the nose and mouth cavities and the pharynx. The left lung has been removed to reveal the heart and some of its major blood vessels.

D reveals the right side of the heart in the chest cavity.

E shows the central (medial) surfaces of the removed right lung.

F reveals the main airway branches within the right lung.

G shows a vertical (sagittal) section through the tissue of the right lung.

1 Hyoid bone
2 Thyroid cartilage
3 Inferior constrictor
 muscle
4 Cricopharyngeus
 muscle
5 Accessory muscles
 from cricoid cartilage
6 Trachea
7 Clavicle
8 Sternum
9 Xiphoid process
10 Cervical vertebrae
11 First rib
12 Scapula
13 Acromion (of scapula)
14 Glenoid fossa (of
 scapula)
15 Costal cartilages
16 Intercostal muscles
17 Pleural reflection
18 Upper surface of
 diaphragm
19 Lateral surfaces of left
 lung

A

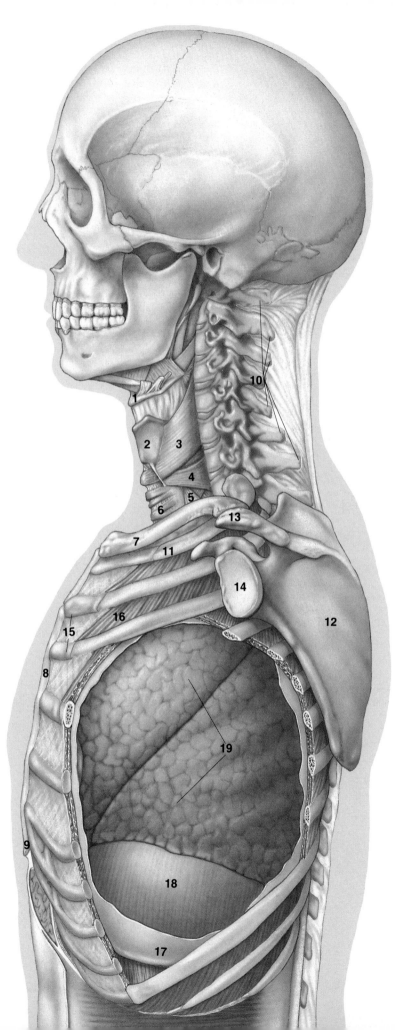

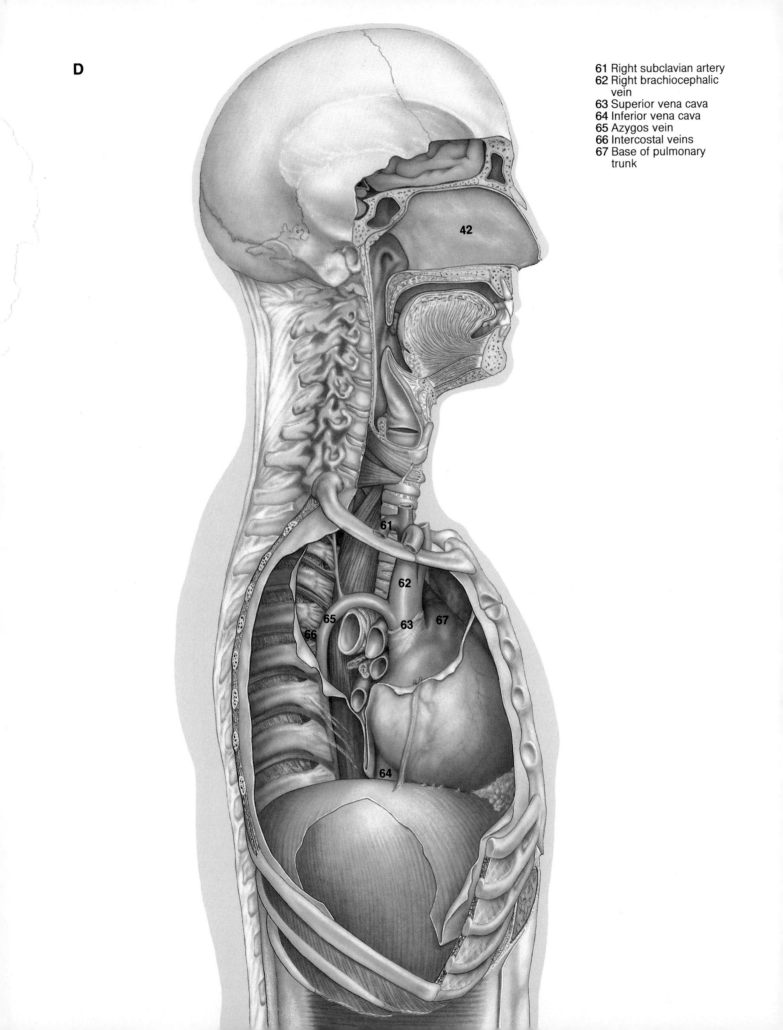

D

61 Right subclavian artery
62 Right brachiocephalic
   vein
63 Superior vena cava
64 Inferior vena cava
65 Azygos vein
66 Intercostal veins
67 Base of pulmonary
   trunk

42 Nasal septum
43 Hard and soft palates
44 Tongue
45 Pharyngeal tonsil
46 Palatine tonsil
47 Epiglottis
48 Esophaghus
49 Thymus
50 Heart with pericardium
51 Aortic arch
52 Descending aorta
53 Left brachiocephalic
   vein
54 Left subclavian artery
55 Left common carotid
   artery
56 Ligamentum arteriosum
57 Mediastinal fatty tissues
58 Thoracic vertebrae
59 Larynx with vocal
   chords
60 Conchae/nasal
   turbinates

C

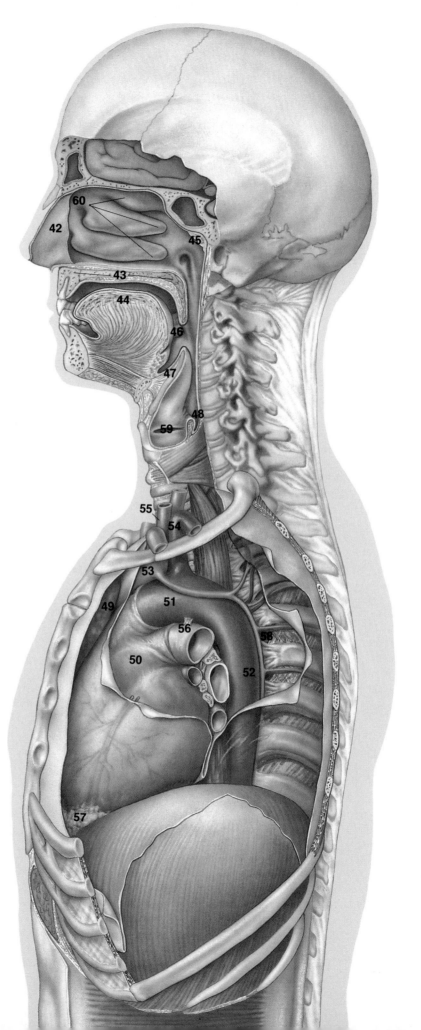

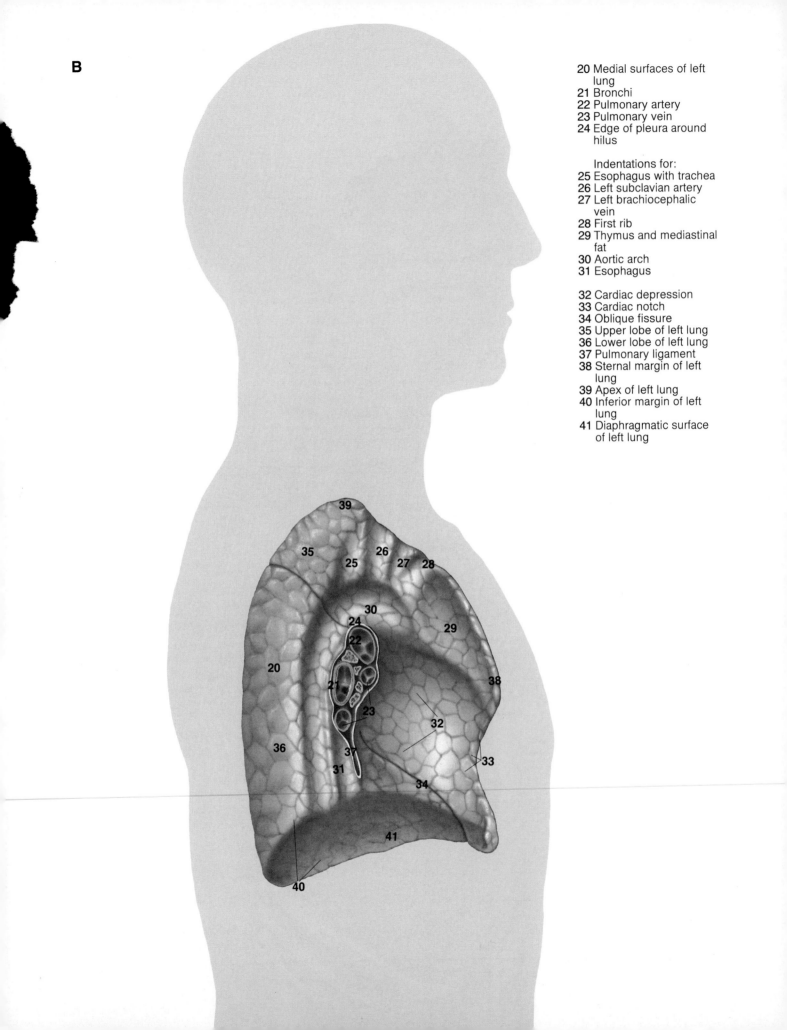

B

20 Medial surfaces of left lung
21 Bronchi
22 Pulmonary artery
23 Pulmonary vein
24 Edge of pleura around hilus

Indentations for:
25 Esophagus with trachea
26 Left subclavian artery
27 Left brachiocephalic vein
28 First rib
29 Thymus and mediastinal fat
30 Aortic arch
31 Esophagus

32 Cardiac depression
33 Cardiac notch
34 Oblique fissure
35 Upper lobe of left lung
36 Lower lobe of left lung
37 Pulmonary ligament
38 Sternal margin of left lung
39 Apex of left lung
40 Inferior margin of left lung
41 Diaphragmatic surface of left lung

68 Upper lobe of right lung
69 Middle lobe of right lung
70 Lower lobe of right lung
71 Horizontal fissure
72 Oblique fissure

Indentations for:
73 Esophagus
74 Trachea
75 Right subclavian artery
76 Right brachiocephalic vein
77 Superior vena cava
78 Inferior vena cava
79 Azygos vein

80 Inferior margin of right lung
81 Sternal margin of right lung
82 Pulmonary ligament
83 Apex of right lung
84 Diaphragmatic surface of right lung
85 Cardiac depression
86 Indentation for thymus and mediastinal fat

E

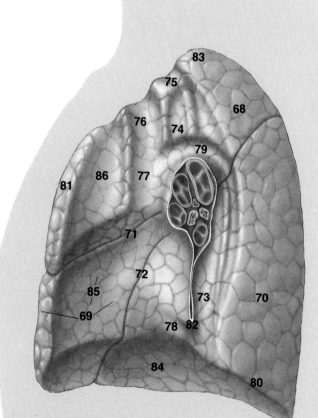

F

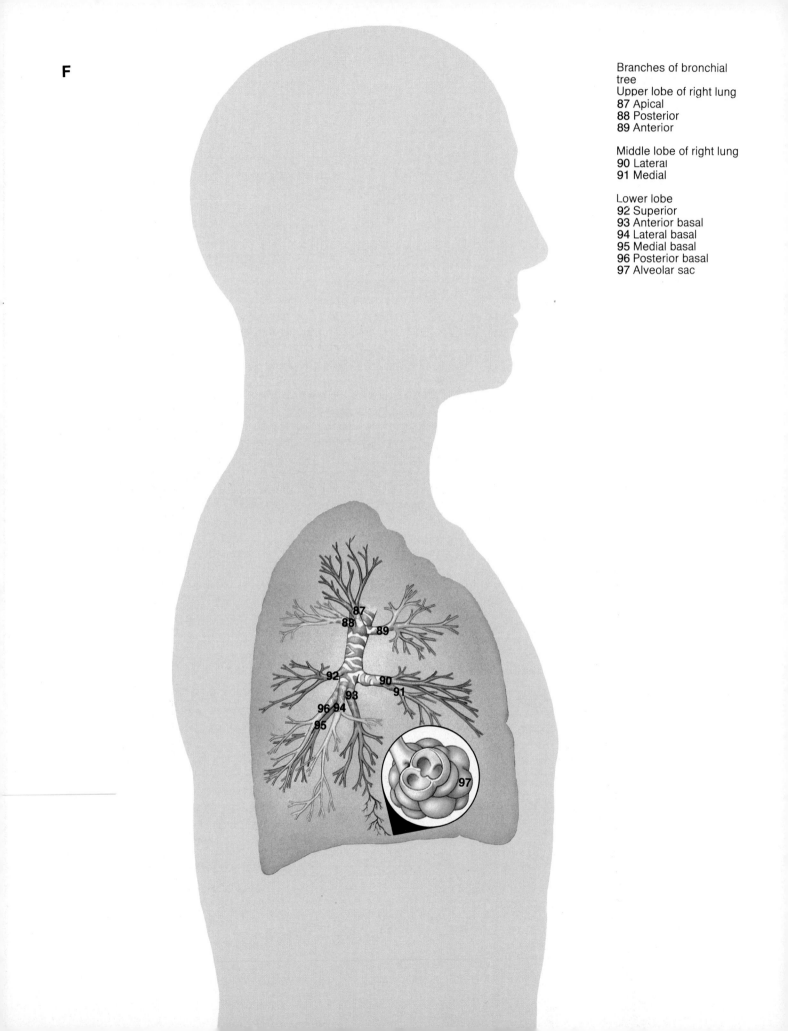

Branches of bronchial
tree
Upper lobe of right lung
87 Apical
88 Posterior
89 Anterior

Middle lobe of right lung
90 Lateral
91 Medial

Lower lobe
92 Superior
93 Anterior basal
94 Lateral basal
95 Medial basal
96 Posterior basal
97 Alveolar sac

98 Cut blood vessels,
    bronchi, bronchioles
99 Pleura

68

98

69

70

99

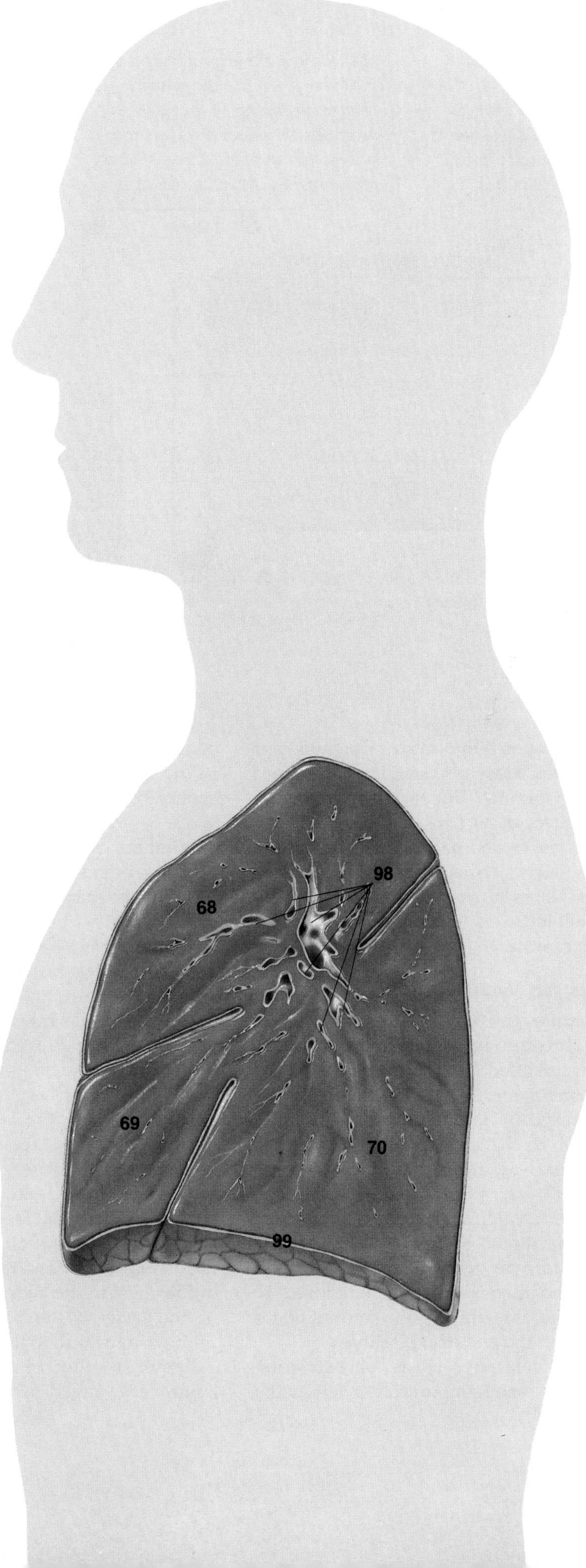

The amount of air breathed in and out of the lungs can be measured by spirometry, among other methods. The patient breathes into and out of a vessel suspended in water from a pulley. The pulley is attached to a pen which marks any movement on a revolving drum. As the patient breathes in, the air in the vessel decreases, the vessel sinks, and the pen records an upward line, showing an increase in the volume of air in the chest. With the out breath, the vessel rises and the pen makes a downward line, showing a decrease in the volume of air in the chest. Vital capacity and tidal volume can both be assessed by this means.

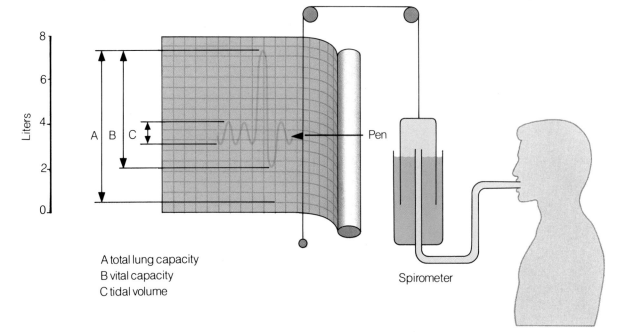

A total lung capacity
B vital capacity
C tidal volume

Pen

Spirometer

Sit down and count the number of breaths you take in one minute. Most adults will breathe about fourteen times a minute, with each breath moving some 500 milliliters of air (the tidal volume). The total volume of air moved per minute (the minute volume) is, therefore, about seven liters, enabling some 1,750 milliliters of oxygen to enter the body and 1,600 milliliters of carbon dioxide to be removed each minute.

Lung Volumes and Ventilation

Most lung volumes can be measured by asking a volunteer to breathe into and out of an air-containing jar inverted over water — a device known as a spirometer. The movements of the spirometer, caused by the volunteer's breathing, are marked on a chart. Volumes that can be measured in this way are the tidal volume, the maximum breath in (tidal volume plus the inspiratory reserve volume), which is about three liters, and the maximum breath out (tidal volume plus the expiratory reserve volume), about one liter. Indirect techniques must be employed to measure the residual volume — the amount of gas left in the lungs at the end of expiration.

This residual volume consists of two components: first, the small amount of air left in the contracted alveoli, and, second, the air remaining in the air-conducting tubes (trachea, bronchi and bronchioles). The second volume is the "dead space" — air that fills the airways during each respiration cycle. It is not available for the real business of gas exchange in the alveoli, hence the term "dead space."

Air that is breathed in is not distributed absolutely evenly throughout the lungs, and its actual dispersal can be measured using xenon which has been made radioactive. A volunteer takes in a single breath of air containing a small amount of the radioactively labeled gas. Wherever the air goes in the lungs, the radioactive xenon goes too, mixed with air, and its presence can be detected outside the body by sensitive scanning apparatus. Thus the pattern of radioactivity revealed by the scanner mirrors the distribution of air in the lungs. Studies using this scanning technique show that there is less air at the top of the lungs than at the bottom and that, if the person lies flat on his or her back, the gradient is from the front of the chest to the back, rather than from the apex of the lung to the base. These differences are thought to be due to the effect of gravity.

Early in the twentieth century, scientific controversy raged as to whether oxygen simply

In a test to discover the distribution of air through the lungs, the patient breathes air containing radioactive material. The presence of the radioactivity in the lungs can be detected by scanning apparatus (right) *showing how the inhaled air has been distributed. Lung function during activity can be tested by an analyzer linked to an exercise machine. Changes in the breathing pattern as exercise progresses are recorded by the machine.*

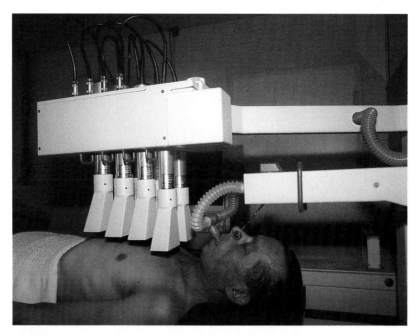

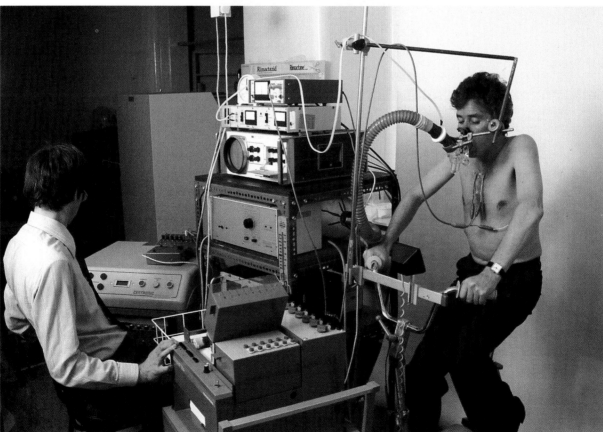

diffused across the alveolar membrane or whether a mechanism existed by which oxygen was actively secreted across into the blood. Supporters of the active secretion theory eventually conceded that oxygen diffuses into the blood capillaries of the lungs and that this process is subject to Fick's Law.

The Law of Diffusion

This law states that the rate of transfer of gas through a sheet of tissue is inversely proportional to the thickness of the tissue and proportional to the tissue area and the difference in gas concentration between the two sides. The thickness of the tissue is obviously crucial. If four people hold the corners of a dry bed sheet while a bucket of water is thrown over it, the water seeps through to the other side immediately. If they then hold a number of dry sheets and repeat the experiment, the water seeps through much more slowly.

In the context of oxygen diffusion from alveoli to capillaries, Fick's Law has a number of obvious implications. Expansion of alveolar volume increases the diffusion area and increases the oxygen transport rate. Potentially, an increase in the thickness of the alveolus wall will decrease the diffusion rate; and the greater the difference in oxygen concentration between the air and the blood, the quicker oxygen will move from alveolus to capillary, or equilibrate.

Also important is the nature of the specific gas, for both the size of its molecules and their solubility will determine the rate of diffusion of a gas. Carbon dioxide, for example, diffuses about twenty times faster than oxygen because, although they have similar molecular weights, carbon dioxide is much more soluble than oxygen.

In each circulation of the blood, a red blood corpuscle is in the pulmonary capillaries for about three-quarters of a second, allowing plenty of time for oxygen to diffuse across from the alveolus and combine with hemoglobin in the red cells. In fact, the rate of oxygen uptake by hemoglobin is one of the limiting factors of oxygen transport. The lung has a large reserve for diffusion and, in normal circumstances, the oxygen concentration in the capillaries when the blood leaves the alveoli is almost identical to that within the alveolus itself. In some situations, however, diffusing capacity

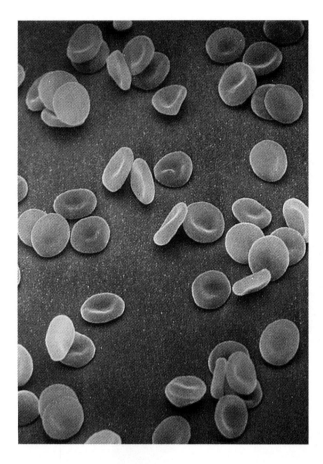

Hemoglobin, contained in the disklike red blood cells (here highly magnified), carries oxygen to all parts of the body. Red blood cells make up about 45 percent of the blood and are the most numerous cells in the body.

becomes limited. During exercise, the blood flows much faster, and the time it spends in the pulmonary system is reduced by two-thirds. In a normal lung, there is sufficient capacity to cope with this, but, in conditions such as fibrosing alveolitis, where the delicate air–blood interface is altered by deposits of fibrous material, there is a limitation of diffusion and oxygenation is reduced.

Diffusion can also be stressed, or limited, by breathing low concentrations of oxygen, either deliberately at normal altitudes or by going to a high altitude, where the pressure of air is much lower and thus the driving force, the concentration gradient, is also lower. Altitude alone causes diffusion limitation, but difficulties occur much earlier under conditions of exercise when there is less time for efficient oxygen transfer to take place. Carbon dioxide diffuses much more readily than oxygen, with rarely, if ever, any limitation.

Blood Flow through the Lungs

A single pump, the heart, drives the two separate blood circulation systems in the body. The circulation to the lungs, the pulmonary circulation, is a relatively low-pressure system, fed with blood from the right side of the heart. The circulation to the rest of the body, the systemic circulation, is a higher-pressure system, supplied via the left side of the heart. The right and left sides of the heart each receive blood and pump it out again. The right and left atria (the upper chambers of the heart) beat together first, pumping the blood into the ventricles, which beat a fraction of a second later.

The course of oxygenated blood through the left side of the heart and on a complete circulation can be followed. The left ventricle, which has a thick muscular wall to power its high-pressure pumping activity, receives from the lungs oxygenated blood that has flowed from the pulmonary veins to the left atrium. The ventricle pumps this blood out into the aorta — the main artery from the heart. A large vessel with a thick muscular wall, the aorta has, on average, an internal pressure of 120 mm Hg during systole — the contraction phase of the left ventricle — and of about 80 mm Hg during diastole — the relaxation phase. These pressure readings approximate to those given by the physician when your blood pressure is taken and may vary up or

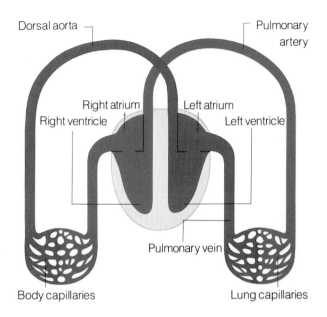

The relationship of the two circulatory systems of the body, the systemic and the pulmonary, is shown in this schematic diagram. The right side of the heart pumps blood to the lungs where it is oxygenated. The oxygenated blood then flows through the pulmonary veins to the left side of the heart, and from there is pumped to every part of the body. In the diagram, red denotes oxygenated blood, blue, deoxygenated.

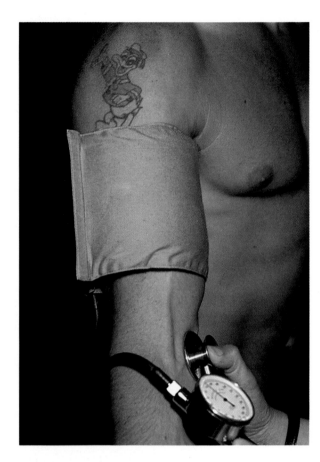

To enable it to circulate around the body, oxygenated blood is pumped out from the heart under considerable pressure. This can be measured by wrapping a cuff around the upper arm and inflating it to a pressure that stops the flow of blood through the artery. As the cuff slowly deflates, the pressure reading of the return of the flow is the peak, or systolic pressure. After further deflation, the lowest, or diastolic, pressure can be read. An average reading for a young adult would be a systolic, or highest, pressure of 120 mm Hg, and a diastolic, or lowest, of 80 mm Hg.

down for a number of reasons, including disease. A value in "mm Hg" means that the pressure has been expressed in terms of millimeters of mercury (the chemical symbol for mercury is Hg). The pressure is defined as that which could support a column of mercury of a particular height. Thus a pressure of 10 mm Hg could support a 10 millimeter column of mercury.

The Pulmonary Pump

The aorta divides into a series of arteries, and the blood flows through these to the arterioles and capillaries until eventually the life-giving oxygen is transferred to all the cells of the body. It is while the blood is in the capillaries that it becomes somewhat darker in color as the oxygen separates from the hemoglobin molecule. Here, too, the gaseous waste product of the cells, carbon dioxide, is picked up.

The blood then returns via the systemic veins to the right atrium of the heart. The pressure of the blood arriving at the heart from the veins is low, about 10 mm Hg, and it is this deoxygenated blood that the heart will pump through the lungs to pick up more oxygen and start the cycle again. The right atrium contracts, and the blood is passed through a three-leafed heart valve, the tricuspid valve, to the right ventricle. There is little increase in pressure at this point. As the pump for the pulmonary circulation, the right ventricle has a muscular wall — not as thick as that of the left ventricle since it has only to pump the blood through one organ, the lung, at relatively low pressure. In fact, the pressure in the main pulmonary artery during systole of the right ventricle is about 25 mm Hg and only about 8 mm Hg during diastole. From the right ventricle, the blood is pumped through the pulmonary valve into the pulmonary artery, which divides into two arteries, one going to the left lung and one to the right lung.

Clearly, the volume of blood pumped from the right ventricle every minute must be the same as that pumped from the left. At rest, this is about 5 liters a minute, although it can increase to 25 liters a minute during vigorous exercise. The quantity of blood in the pulmonary circulation at any moment is 10 to 20 percent of the total volume, that is, half to one liter. Usually the five liters of blood pumping

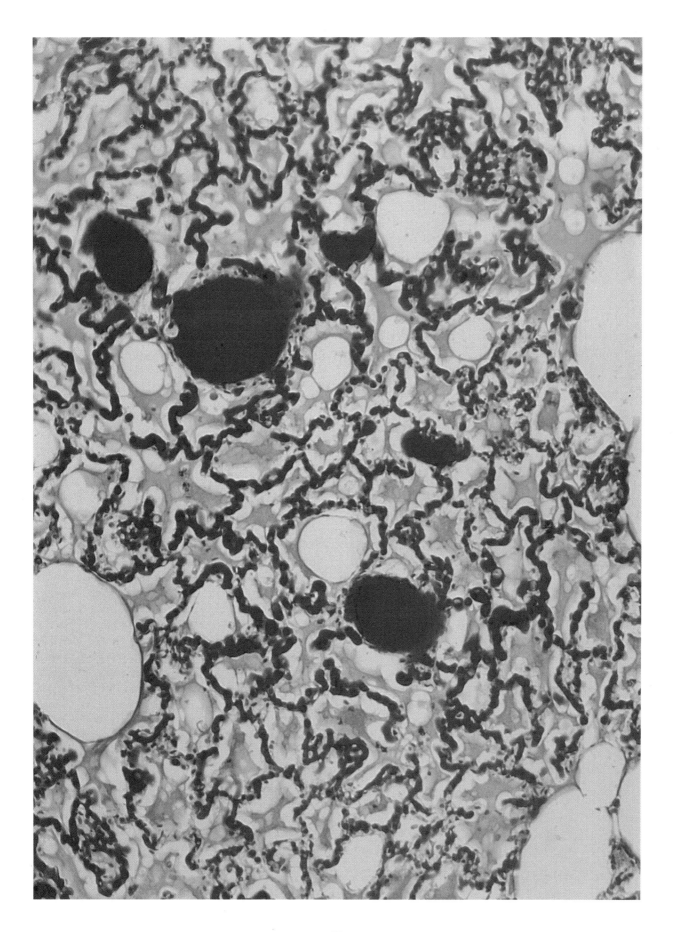

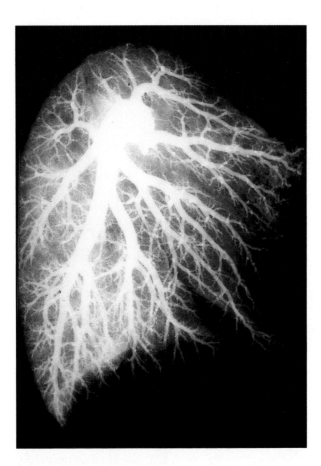

Resembling a mass of fine plant roots, a complex arterial system supplies blood to the lung. The tubes have been made visible in this X ray picture by injecting an X ray opaque medium into the blood vessels.

around the pulmonary circulation is divided almost equally between the two lungs. Gravity has its effect, however, and if a person lies on his side, the lower, dependent lung will have an increased percentage of the blood coming from the heart.

The pulmonary arteries branch successively in a similar manner to the bronchi and follow a similar course, eventually dividing and providing blood to the capillary bed. The rich network of capillaries has a surface area similar to that of the alveoli, surrounding and bathing their walls and resembling a sheet of flowing blood rather than individual segments. Narrow and thin-walled, the capillaries allow little more than a single red blood cell to flow through at a time. Gas transfer occurs in the capillary bed, and blood flowing out is high in oxygen, low in carbon dioxide. The oxygenated blood flows through a system of small veins, or venules, which join to form the pulmonary veins. These unite to form one large vein from each lung, which also join and enter the left side of the heart at the left atrium. Having returned to the heart, the oxygenated blood is now pumped around the body again in the continuing cycle of life.

Shunted Blood

Not all of the blood returning to the left atrium is fully oxygenated, and some blood that flows into it has not passed through the lung; such blood is known as shunted blood. A normal shunt can occur in several ways. A certain amount of blood from the systemic circulation supplies oxygenated blood to the bronchi and most of this returns via the normal venous system to the right atrium. Some, however, joins up with the pulmonary veins and is returned to the left atrium. Another route by which deoxygenated blood finds its way into the left side of the heart is through the direct drainage of a small amount of blood from the coronary circulation into the cavity of the left ventricle. People with congenital heart disease may have abnormal connections between the right and left sides of the heart so that quantities of deoxygenated blood from the pulmonary system return directly to the systemic circulation. This is a right-to-left shunt.

Blood is unevenly distributed throughout the lungs. In a standing person, for example, there is less blood at the top of the lungs than at the bottom.

By using a modified version of the radioactive xenon described earlier for measuring air distribution, the distribution of blood can be measured. Radioactive gas is dissolved in water and the substance injected into a vein, thus radioactively labeling the blood. The blood containing the radioactive xenon reaches the lungs and diffuses across into the gas inside the lungs. Radiation counters positioned over the chest wall then measure the amount and dispersal of radioactivity. Where the counter registers a high degree of radioactivity, a great deal of blood has passed through that part of the lungs. Where there is no radioactivity, no blood has passed through that area. The blood flow gradually decreases on moving up the lung until, at the top, or apex, almost no blood flows at all.

If the subject lies down, the blood is redistributed so that the apex receives the same amount as the base, but the back receives more than the front. Upside down, the apex has a higher blood flow than the base, an effect due, in part, to gravity. In the upright position, blood has to be pumped more to reach the top of the lung, and the pressure in the pulmonary circulation is not high.

There is a particular mechanism for preserving blood flow through the lungs (perfusion) in adverse circumstances. Known as hypoxic pulmonary vasoconstriction, the mechanism operates in such a way that if the amount of oxygen in the alveoli of a particular lung region decreases (hypoxia), the blood flow to that region is reduced by tightening up the muscles of the arteriolar wall (vasoconstriction). Blood can then be diverted to a region where the amount of oxygen is greater. This response can be important in illness because it keeps blood away from blocked-off areas of the lung such as can occur in pneumonia.

At high altitudes, where oxygen pressure is lower, a generalized hypoxic vasoconstriction may occur. The resistance of the pulmonary arteries is thus increased, so the heart has to pump harder to get the blood through the pulmonary circulation.

The workings of hypoxic pulmonary vasoconstriction are still not fully understood; it is known, however, that it does not depend on control from the nervous system. Experiments on lungs removed from animals show that the mechanism is still intact even without the nervous system.

Much of contemporary understanding of lung physiology comes from the work of Californian physiologist J. B. West. One of his major areas of research has been an investigation of the way in which ventilation and blood flow match one another. If they matched perfectly, there would be no discrepancy between the oxygen in the lungs and the oxygen in the blood. However, the tension of oxygen in the blood of the pulmonary veins is not the same as that in the lungs. In normal people there is little difference between the two, but in those suffering from lung disease, the differences may become exaggerated and cause the blood to be low in oxygen.

The Control of Respiration

Inherently rhythmic, the heart keeps on beating even if all the nerves supplying it are cut. The muscles that effect ventilation have no such property, and if the nerves supplying them are severed, respiration cannot continue.

Although we breathe automatically, without giving it a thought, we can exert some control over our own respiration. The normal adult rate of respiration is fourteen breaths a minute. Now see how many breaths you can take in one minute, breathing as fast as you can. It will be considerably more. Breathe normally for a minute or two, then stop breathing and time yourself while holding your breath. Take ten really deep breaths and hold your breath again and you will find that you can hold it for longer. This is because the ten really deep breaths have "blown off" the carbon dioxide from the lungs and the blood and an increase in the concentration of carbon dioxide in the blood is one of the main internal stimuli to the brain to increase respiration. The control mechanism has to operate with considerable sensitivity as the carbon dioxide concentration changes are never more than 3 mm Hg, whatever the exercise being undertaken.

The brain centers controlling respiration are situated in the brain stem, the part of the brain just above the spinal column. Chemoreceptors in the brain stem are sensitive to the chemical composition of the fluid surrounding them — in this instance their sensitivity is to carbon dioxide. The chemoreceptors are not actually in contact with

John Bernard West

Master of Lung Physiology

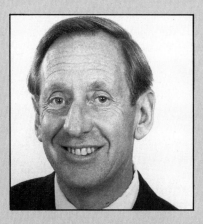

In the spring of 1961, an exercise bicycle was assembled on the snowbound slopes of Mount Makalu, some 24,400 feet up in the Himalayas. One by one, members of the Himalayan Scientific and Mountaineering Expedition, led by Sir Edmund Hillary, climbed onto the bicycle to have their exercise performance closely monitored by a team of scientists. One of those scientists investigating the effects of altitude on the human body, particularly on lung function, was physiologist John Bernard West.

Born in 1928 in Adelaide, Australia, West obtained his medical degree at the university there in 1952; he then moved to London, England to study for a Ph.D. His interest in the physiology of the lungs, in particular, the exchange of gases, was stimulated by the development, by K. T. Fowler of the Hammersmith Hospital, London, England, of the respiratory mass spectrometer. This machine identifies and measures the amount of substances, such as oxygen, in the lungs.

When a radioactive oxygen was produced in the late 1950s, John West saw its potential for use in experiments on the pulmonary exchange of gases and developed an interest in the distribution of blood flow in the lung. By asking volunteers to inhale the gas and then scanning the distribution of radioactivity in the lungs, he and his team were able to obtain measurements of blood flow and ventilation in the human lung.

Until this time, accurate information on ventilation and perfusion in the lungs was available only from analysis of expired gas and arterial blood. Now abnormalities in the ventilation–perfusion relationship could be localized by use of this revolutionary technique.

Since that time further techniques for scanning the entire lung have been developed. For example, in 1974 John West, with P. D. Wagner and H. A. Saltzman, perfected a multiple inert gas technique which gives information about the complete and continuous distribution of gas ventilation and blood perfusion throughout the lungs. Not only do such techniques reveal much about the function and fine tuning of the lungs, they also help with the diagnosis of pulmonary disease.

Continuing his studies on lung function in extreme conditions, of which the Himalayan experiments were part, John West spent a year at NASA's Ames Research Center, Moffett Field, California. Here he worked on the effects on the lungs of weightlessness in space. He is currently Principal Investigator of an experiment to measure the effects of space travel on pulmonary function in astronauts, an experiment scheduled to fly in Spacelab 4 in 1985. Among the many tests to be carried out will be experiments to study the alterations in the distribution of ventilation and blood flow in astronauts while in conditions of weightlessness.

Dr. West is now settled permanently in the U.S.A. and is Professor of Medicine and Physiology at the University of California, San Diego. Much of his time is dedicated to teaching, and he has published books on respiratory physiology used by students all over the world. His influential achievements in the field of physiology were justly rewarded when he was elected President of the American Physiological Society in July 1984.

blood but with cerebrospinal fluid, a clear fluid bathing the brain. Carbon dioxide diffuses into this fluid from the blood, however, and the concentrations are the same. When there is an increase in carbon dioxide at the brain stem chemoreceptors, messages are sent via the spinal column to the nerves supplying the muscles of the diaphragm. Peripheral chemoreceptors in the bloodstream, the arch of the aorta and the carotid arteries also respond to carbon dioxide and send messages to the brain when they detect alterations in its levels. They are, however, much less important in the control of ventilation than are the central chemoreceptors in the brain.

If the blood is low in oxygen, however, this is sensed exclusively by the peripheral chemoreceptors, since there are no oxygen receptors in the brain. Messages are relayed from these receptors to the receptors in the brain stem, causing an increase in respiratory drive to restore the oxygen level.

Other Functions of the Lungs

Gas exchange is not the sole function of the lungs. In addition to filtering small particles and humidifying, warming or cooling the inspired air, lungs have other ways of contributing to the well-being of the body. Although they cannot deal with large clots, the lungs can filter out many of the small blood clots, or thrombi, that occur in the bloodstream and prevent them from entering the systemic circulation and reaching the brain, heart or other vital organs. The lungs also contain tissues which synthesize such compounds as depalmitoyl lecithin, the phospholipid that is the main component of surfactant.

Lungs have a subsidiary role in the control of the body's blood pressure, too. An inactive hormone, angiotensin I, is produced near the kidneys but converted by an enzyme of the cells of the pulmonary capillaries into the potent hormone angiotensin II. This active hormone causes arteries to constrict, increasing blood pressure. The lungs are a particularly suitable site for such a conversion, since all the blood flow must pass through the lungs in each circulation. As much as a 70 percent conversion of inactive to active hormone takes place in a single passage of blood through the pulmonary capillaries.

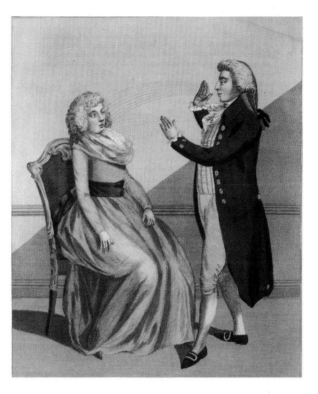

When inducing a state of trance, a hypnotist asks the subject first to take a deep breath and then to continue to breathe quietly and easily. This helps the subject to release tension and accept the trance. While in a trance, the subject's body relaxes, and breathing is slow and regular.

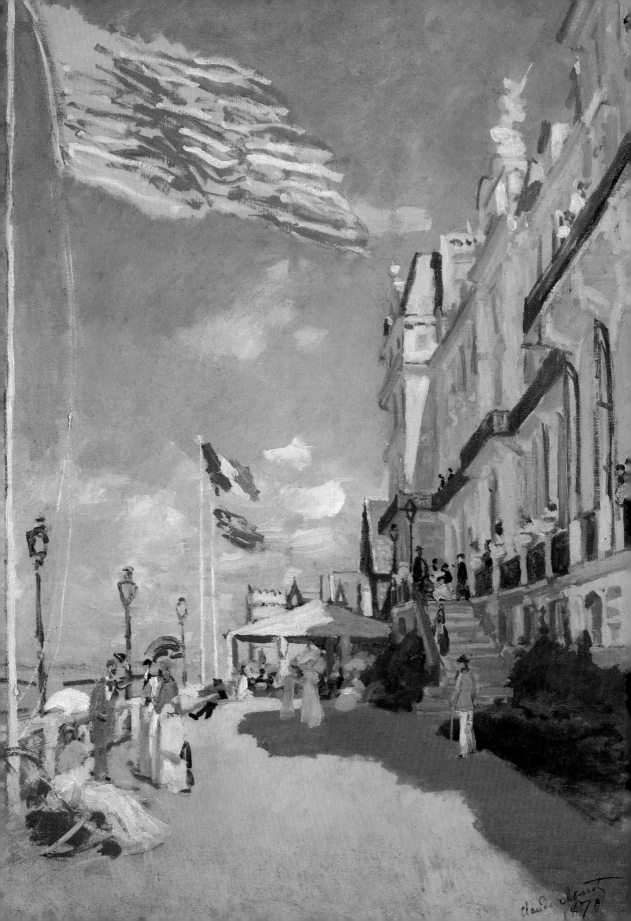

Chapter 4

Faulty Airways

Normal breathing depends on the efficient operation of the respiratory pump (the muscles of respiration and the bony thorax), the conducting airways, and the diffusion of oxygen and carbon dioxide across the alveolar-capillary unit. But what happens to respiration if the pump slows down or operates inefficiently; if the conducting airways are abnormal due to lung disease or injury; or if the diffusion process is disrupted by lung disease?

The system can go wrong in other ways too. Normally, the pulmonary blood vessels deliver blood poor in oxygen from the heart to the lungs for carbon dioxide to be removed and oxygen replenished, and they carry freshly oxygenated blood away from the lungs to the heart from where it is pumped throughout the body. In some diseases, blood actually bypasses the lungs and never receives oxygen. In others, part of the lung is so diseased that no oxygen gets into the blood passing through that section of the lung.

Finally, the effects of gravity, small in normal lungs, are increased by most lung diseases. Gravity affects the distribution of ventilation and blood flow in the lungs, creating a mismatching of these processes. More blood flow goes to the bottom of the lung, and, to a lesser extent, more ventilation occurs there as well. Increased mismatching of ventilation and blood flow due to lung disease is one of the most important causes of low oxygen levels in patients.

To examine these malfunctions of the respiratory system in detail, it is pertinent to look first at the effects of the slowing down or inefficient operation of the respiratory pump. A reduction in the volume of fresh air going into the lungs and alveoli is termed hypoventilation. If the functions of the body that require oxygen continue at the same rate despite this reduction, the level of oxygen that can be measured in the blood will invariably be lowered. The other effect of hypoventilation is that

In nineteenth-century Europe it was fashionable to spend time at seaside resorts to "take the air." City dwellers promenaded, enjoying relief from the new phenomenon of industrial pollution. In Claude Monet's painting L'Hôtel des Roches Noires à Trouville *(1870), he conveys a vivid feeling of such seaside freshness, with the wide airy sky and fluffy clouds. Even if the benefits of "sea air" were exaggerated, at least people felt it was doing them good.*

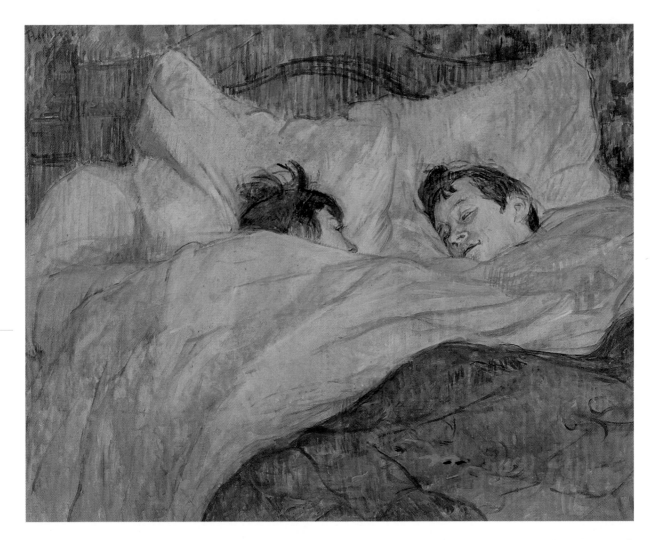

if carbon dioxide is being produced by metabolism in the cells of the body at a constant rate, and less air is moving into and out of the lungs, less carbon dioxide will be removed from the blood. If measured, the carbon dioxide level in the blood will be higher than normal.

Some degree of hypoventilation occurs in a number of normal situations, unrelated to disease. During sleep, for instance, respiration becomes slower, each breath may be less deep, and the overall amount of ventilation is reduced. The lowering of the blood oxygen level and the elevation of the blood carbon dioxide level during sleep is not ordinarily significant. If hypoventilation is marked, however, dangerously low oxygen levels can result.

What causes the respiratory pump drastically to decrease its level of function? Hypoventilation is commonly caused by diseases outside the lungs and, in fact, the lungs themselves are usually normal. There are four major reasons for hypoventilation: abnormalities of respiratory control;

malfunction of the respiratory muscles; chest wall disease and obesity.

Abnormalities of Respiratory Control

If the drive to breathe, which is controlled by the brain, is depressed, the pump will slow down or stop — an exaggeration of what happens during sleep. General anesthesia causes the brain to go into an extremely deep sleep; the respiratory center of the brain is depressed and no longer sends nerve signals to the muscles of the respiratory system to contract and move the pump. When this "deep sleep" is induced by anesthesia, the respiratory pump function must be taken over by a machine pump to support ventilation.

Certain drugs, too, such as barbiturate sleeping pills or narcotic pain relievers, can depress the respiratory center in the brain and must, therefore, be used with extreme caution. Overdoses of these agents can be fatal because they stop the operation of the respiratory pump by turning off its main switch in the brain.

In one rare disorder of the brain's respiratory center, the automatic stimulus to breathe is lost, causing hypoventilation. Known as "Ondine's curse," the disorder is named after the myth of Ondine the mermaid. Ondine's curse was that if a human were to fall in love with her, he would lose the ability for automatic activity. If he did not remember to breathe voluntarily, he would be unable to do so spontaneously. Patients suffering from "Ondine's curse" often experience overall hypoventilation and pauses in respiration.

Problems with Respiratory Muscles

If the respiratory center is active, but the nerves that conduct the signals in the spinal cord and to the respiratory muscles are disrupted, hypoventilation results. This reduction in breathing efficiency can also be caused by diseases affecting the strength and efficiency of muscle contraction.

Polio victims, for example, because of damage to the nerve fibers that control the muscles of respiration, do not have the muscle power to work the respiratory pump. The artificial, or iron, lung was developed in the 1950s to replace the patient's own failing respiratory muscles. The patient lay in the tank, and negative pressure around the chest caused it to expand and air to enter the lungs.

Other diseases affecting nerves and muscles, such as amyotrophic lateral sclerosis, or Lou Gehrig's disease, can cause hypoventilation in the same way and, eventually, respiratory failure.

Chest Wall Disease

Impaired ventilation can be caused by a distorted chest skeleton, resulting from disease or injury. For air to enter the lungs after the brain initiates the ventilatory drive and the respiratory muscles contract, the thorax must be expandable, and it is this enlargement of the thoracic volume which creates the negative pressure that brings air into the lungs. Certain skeletal diseases can result in a distorted chest which will not expand appropriately; one example is kyphoscoliosis, the disease suffered by the "Hunchback of Nôtre Dame."

In addition to being able to expand, the bony thorax must be stable. If it collapsed during respiratory muscular contraction, thoracic volume would not change, and negative pressure would

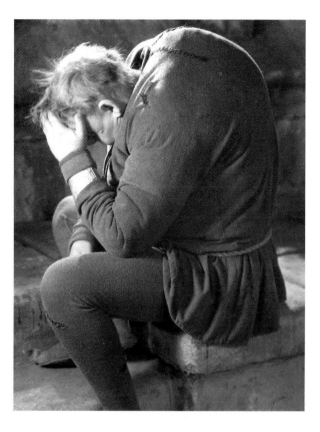

The Hunchback of Nôtre Dame suffered from kyphoscoliosis, an exaggeration of the curve of the spine both sideways and outward. The disease is generally accompanied by respiratory problems, since the lungs cannot expand properly in the distorted chest and capacity is therefore reduced.

not develop. Multiple broken ribs can cause this type of chest wall instability — the so-called "flail chest" — and lead to hypoventilation.

The Pickwickian Syndrome

Severely obese people may suffer from hypoventilation. This tendency is often referred to as the "Pickwickian syndrome" after Joe, the fat boy, a character in Charles Dickens's *Pickwick Papers* who was obese, excessively sleepy during the day and snored heavily.

> " 'Damn that boy,' said the old gentleman, 'he's gone to sleep again.' 'Very extraordinary boy, that,' said Mr. Pickwick, 'does he always sleep in this way?' 'Sleep,' said the old gentleman, 'he's always asleep. Goes on errands fast asleep, and snores as he waits on table.'
>
> The fat boy rose, opened his eyes, swallowed the huge piece of pie he had been in the act of masticating when he last fell asleep, and slowly obeyed his master's orders — gloating languidly over the remains of the feast as he removed the plates, and deposited them in the hamper. . . ."

The fat boy probably suffered from hypoventilation because so much weight had to be moved with each breath. Indeed, Dickens is generally acknowledged to be the first to give a detailed description of this obesity-linked breathing disorder. In addition to the increased workload for the respiratory system, Pickwickian patients are likely to have abnormalities in their central nervous system control of respiration. Their heavy snoring is often associated with apnea, or the cessation of breathing, during sleep. Their sleep is disrupted and fragmented, thus they are always sleepy.

Hypoventilation then, the reduction in the amount of air going to, and being removed from, the alveoli, can have profound effects on gas exchange. As was mentioned earlier, in most instances the lungs are actually normal, and if extra oxygen is provided to the hypoventilating patient, the low level of oxygen can easily be raised.

Oxygen in the alveoli must traverse the blood–gas barrier of the alveolar cell and capillary membrane and combine with hemoglobin, within red blood cells, to be transported to the body tissues.

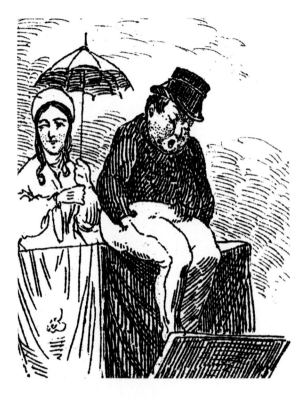

Joe, the fat boy, a character in Charles Dickens's novel Pickwick Papers, *appeared to suffer from the condition now known, in his honor, as the Pickwickian syndrome. Obese people may have breathing difficulties, first, simply because so much weight has to be moved with each breath, and second, because their upper airways easily become obstructed at pharynx level. The latter is particularly likely to occur during sleep, hence the patient wakes many times and, as a result, like Joe, is constantly sleepy.*

If the walls of the alveoli become injured and thickened or if the overall surface area of the blood-gas barrier is reduced, diffusion can become more difficult. Some primary lung diseases result in thickened alveolar-capillary membranes due to alveolar injury, and the slowing of diffusion caused by this contributes to abnormalities in gas exchange in such patients. Sometimes this impairment of diffusion can be brought about by exercise. It is common, for example, for patients with diffusion defects to complain of shortness of breath when exercising but to be quite comfortable at rest. The explanation for this pattern is that exercise increases blood flow through the lungs, and, as its rate of flow through the pulmonary capillaries increases, the amount of time the blood maintains contact with the alveolar gas decreases. If the alveolar membrane is abnormal and more time is, therefore, needed for oxygen to traverse it, there may not be enough time for sufficient diffusion to take place during the increased blood flow of exercise. In addition, during exercise more oxygen is used and demand is higher.

Impairment of Diffusion

In the normal alveolar-capillary unit, delicate membranes separate air and blood. In a diseased lung, the alveolar walls are much thicker, and many cells fill the space between the air and blood compartments. Such a lung may also show considerable scarring and increase in fibrous tissue, or fibrosis. Diffusion will be slowed and impaired, particularly when the patient exercises. Oxygen levels will be reduced during exercise, but, unlike patients who suffer from hypoventilation, carbon dioxide retention does not usually develop in these cases. Carbon dioxide is much more soluble than oxygen, so is more readily diffusible.

Diffusion abnormalities are a small contributory factor in the condition of hypoxemia — low levels of oxygen in the blood — in any lung disease in which the alveolar capillary membrane is injured. Diffusion impairment also plays a role in diseases, such as emphysema, in which lung destruction reduces the number of capillaries and, therefore, the capillary surface area for diffusion. Lastly, in patients with a severe reduction in the numbers of red blood cells, diffusion is also impaired.

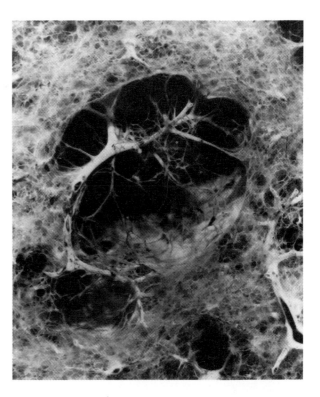

A scanning electron micrograph shows the cut surface of a lung tissue biopsy specimen from a patient suffering from emphysema. It reveals the dramatic disruption of the normal alveolar structure caused by the disease and the consequent enlargement of the air spaces.

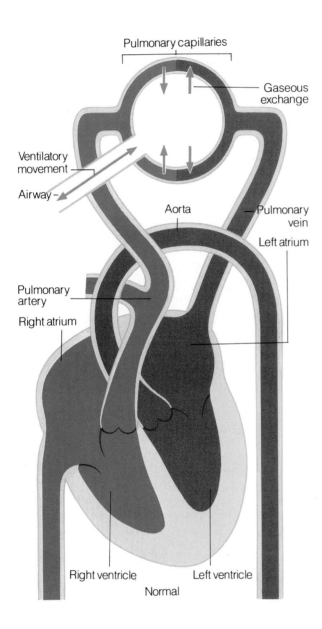

Pulmonary capillaries

Gaseous
exchange

Ventilatory
movement

Airway

Aorta

Pulmonary
vein

Left atrium

Pulmonary
artery

Right atrium

Right ventricle

Left ventricle

Normal

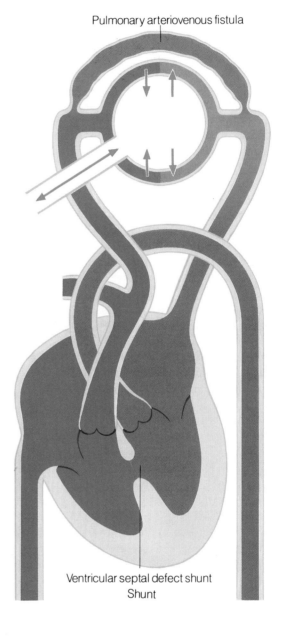

Pulmonary arteriovenous fistula

Ventricular septal defect shunt

Shunt

The normal circulation of the body is contrasted with that occurring as a result of cardiac pulmonary shunts. Abnormal connections between, for example, the ventricles, or the pulmonary artery and vein, can result in blood that has not been properly oxygenated entering the general body circulation. The overall level of blood oxygen is then lowered.

Shunted Blood

In previous chapters it has been noted that not all of the blood flowing from the heart goes through the ventilated portions of the lungs. A small amount, the purpose of which is to supply oxygen and nutrients to the bronchial tubes themselves, goes directly back to the heart, by way of the bronchial circulation to the pulmonary veins, without being reoxygenated. This oxygen-poor blood mixes with the oxygenated blood in the pulmonary veins and lowers the body's overall oxygen level slightly. This is called a shunt — a pattern of blood flow that reaches the arterial system without passing through ventilated regions of the lungs.

In babies born with heart defects, a significant amount of blood can be shunted through the heart or great vessels away from the lungs. These babies are often "blue" because this shunted, oxygen-poor blood significantly lowers their overall blood oxygen level. Shunts can also occur in the lung when an abnormal connection between a pulmonary artery and pulmonary vein has formed — a pulmonary arteriovenous fistula.

When an area of the lung is completely filled with disease, such as pneumonia or pulmonary edema, and no ventilation at all occurs in that area of the lung, the blood passing through it can also be considered to be shunted blood, since it does not come into contact with alveolar gas and become enriched with oxygen.

If blood oxygen has been lowered because of a shunt in the heart, the pulmonary blood vessels or the lung, administering extra oxygen will have no major effect and will not raise the blood oxygen level dramatically. This is because the extra oxygen never comes in contact with the shunted blood.

Mismatching of Ventilation and Blood Flow

The normal lung has some unevenness in the distribution of ventilation and blood flow. When a normal person stands upright, there is more ventilation than blood flow at the top of the lung. In the middle zone, ventilation and blood flow are evenly matched; while at the base of the lung, there is more blood flow than ventilation.

Distribution of ventilation and blood flow is changed dramatically by lung disease. In patients

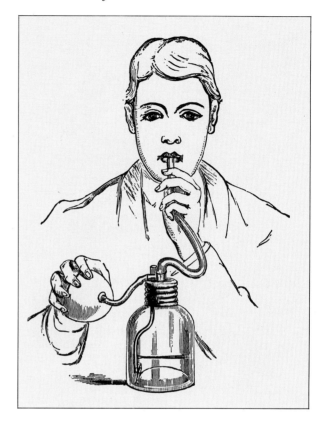

with diseases obstructing the flow of air through the bronchial tubes, or in whom alveoli are destroyed and not properly filled or emptied, areas of the lung previously well ventilated will receive considerably less air due to this obstruction. In contrast, patients with diseases affecting the pulmonary blood vessels, such as pulmonary embolism in which a clot obstructs blood flow to a part of the lung, may have extra areas of the lung where ventilation exceeds the blood flow. Both types of inequality — excess and decreased ventilation in relation to blood flow — can have a significant effect on the function of the lung in its role as exchanger of oxygen and carbon dioxide.

If lung disease is extreme, as in emphysema (in which the alveoli are destroyed), chronic bronchitis, asthma or severe pneumonia, two main gas exchange problems develop. Areas of decreased ventilation in relation to blood flow contribute less well oxygenated blood to the total amount of arterial blood leaving the lung to be pumped to the tissues by the heart. This lowers the overall level of

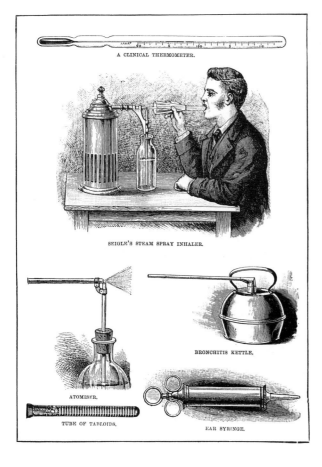

A CLINICAL THERMOMETER.

SEIGLE'S STEAM SPRAY INHALER.

BRONCHITIS KETTLE.

ATOMISER.

TUBE OF TABLOIDS.

EAR SYRINGE.

blood oxygen and is similar to the way in which shunted blood lowers the blood oxygen level.

Areas of excess ventilation in relation to blood flow are areas where ventilation is "wasted" — that is, ventilation to poorly perfused alveoli contributes little or nothing to the oxygenation of the blood. These areas of wasted ventilation or "dead space" do not directly cause low oxygen levels, but the overall level of ventilation must be increased to maintain adequate carbon dioxide elimination. Unequal distribution of ventilation and blood flow is probably the most important and common cause of abnormalities of gas exchange in lung disease.

Types of Respiratory Disease

Most lung diseases can be classified according to the pattern of functional abnormality present. In some patients with lung disease such as asthma or emphysema, the major abnormality in function is that air flow through the conducting airways is limited and obstructed. When a patient with predominantly obstructive lung disease is tested in a pulmonary function laboratory, he or she takes a deep breath to the upper capacity of the lungs, then blows out the air as rapidly and completely as possible. The rate of flow of air out of the lungs is greatly reduced compared to that of a normal individual. A larger than usual volume of air may also remain in the lung: the residual volume. The obstruction of the airways causes this remaining air to be trapped.

Time courses of forced expiration in patients suffering from obstructive and restrictive disease are here compared with that of a normal person. In the patient with obstructive disease, the rate of flow of air out of the lungs is greatly reduced because of the obstruction in the airways, and a larger than usual volume may remain in the lungs. The patient with restrictive disease is unable to take in as much air as the normal person due to the restriction of the lungs, but the rate of flow out of the lungs may be above average.

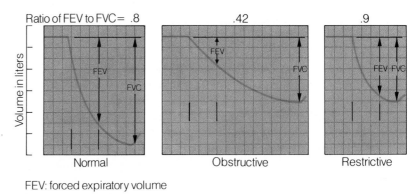

Ratio of FEV to FVC = .8   .42   .9

Volume in liters

Normal   Obstructive   Restrictive

FEV: forced expiratory volume
FVC: forced vital capacity

The other major abnormality found on pulmonary function testing in patients with lung disease is that the volume of air in the lungs is being restricted. When patients with restrictive disease are asked to breathe in and fill their lungs completely, they are unable to take in an adequate volume of air, compared to normal people of the same height and weight. The total lung capacity is reduced, but there is no obstruction of air flow. On expiration, this reduced volume of air leaves the lungs promptly and completely.

Air Flow Obstruction

Any structural change that increases resistance to air flow in the large or small conducting airways can cause obstructive lung disease.

The bronchial tubes themselves may be partially plugged with mucus or other secretions — for example in patients with chronic inflammation and infection in their bronchi. Cigarette smokers who habitually cough and bring up sputum may have chronic bronchitis, and many of their bronchial tubes may be partially obstructed with mucus.

Increased resistance to air flow can also be caused by changes in the wall of the bronchial tubes. In asthma, the muscle in the bronchial wall contracts and goes into spasm during an acute attack. This muscular contraction narrows the diameter of the bronchial tubes and causes the resistance to air flow to increase. Air flow can be severely limited in this way in asthmatics, and, in a serious attack, air

movement may be drastically reduced until this bronchial spasm is relieved. In addition to bronchial muscle contraction and spasm, asthmatics may have swelling of the bronchial walls and excessive mucus production, occasionally leading to bronchial obstruction which further limits air flow.

Air flow obstruction can also be caused by changes in the structure of the lung surrounding the airway. A normal lung has elastic properties, which make it like a "slinky" or a rubber band. When stretched, it tends to recoil or collapse. This tendency of the lung tissue surrounding the airways to elastic recoil exerts a pulling, or traction, effect on the airways, helping to keep them wide open. In addition, elastic recoil of the lung is what drives air out of the alveoli during expiration. In emphysema, some of the lung tissue is destroyed and the elastic recoil tendency reduced, so not only are the airways narrowed but the driving force behind expiration is also reduced.

Effects of Obstruction on Lung Function

The hallmarks of obstructive lung disease are the slowing down of forced expiration due to bronchial obstruction, bronchial spasm and narrowing due to asthma, and the excessive narrowing of the airways during expiration. The last of these is due to the loss of the elastic recoil properties of the surrounding lung. In severe obstructive lung disease, air may be trapped in the lung, leading to a large residual volume after an attempt has been

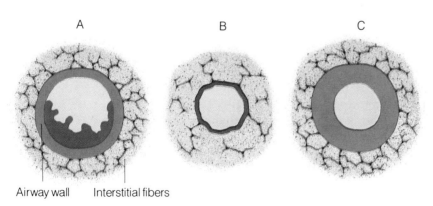

A   B   C

Airway wall   Interstitial fibers

Effects on airways of obstructive lung disease

There are three major ways in which the airways can become blocked in patients suffering from obstructive lung disease. First, the airway may be partially blocked by excessive mucus (A); second, it may become narrowed by loss of traction in the surrounding interstitial fibers (B); third, the wall of the airway may thicken, causing a narrowing of the airway itself (C). In all the effect is the same — the free flow of air is hindered, reducing the efficiency of respiration.

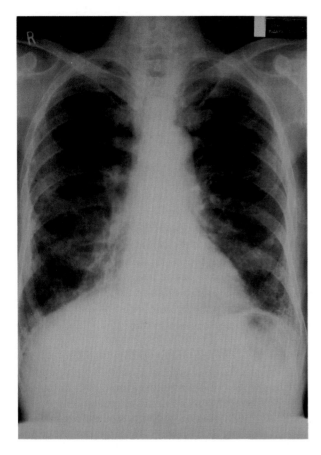

made to exhale totally. This overinflation increases the work that the respiratory muscles must perform to move the respiratory system and reduces the efficiency and capacity of ventilation.

Patients with bronchial obstruction as the primary cause of increased air flow resistance may suffer significantly reduced ventilation even in areas of the lung where blood flow is well preserved. This results in mismatching of ventilation and blood flow, which in turn causes lowering of blood oxygen.

In emphysema patients, lung destruction and loss of supporting lung tissue accounts for air flow obstruction. Lung destruction also reduces the number of pulmonary capillaries, and some regions of the lung will have high ventilation relative to their blood flow. This ventilation is, however, partially wasted.

To compensate for significant areas of the lung in which ventilation is wasted, the respiratory pump must increase its overall level of ventilation to remove all the carbon dioxide produced by cellular metabolism. Late in the disease, however, carbon dioxide retention may develop despite these compensatory efforts.

Restriction of Lung Volume

Changes in the structure of the respiratory system can result from restriction of lung volume. Restriction can be caused by any of three factors: first, disease in the lung itself; second, disease in the covering of the lung — the pleura; and third, disease in the chest wall or muscles of respiration.

In the condition diffuse interstitial fibrosis, for example, the scarring and fibrosis of the lung greatly increases the elastic recoil tendency. The lungs are always tending toward deflation, and, on inflation, they are found to be stiff — their compliance is decreased. This loss of compliance is the cause of restricted, reduced lung volumes in this disease.

Diseases such as sarcoidosis, asbestosis and interstitial pulmonary edema all affect the interstitial areas of the lung — the areas between the alveoli — and, therefore, also result in reduced lung volumes and loss of compliance. In these diseases, however, the airways are usually not involved and may, in fact, be wider in diameter than normal. These dilated small airways, surrounded by scarred, thickened connective tissue, have been likened to a honeycomb in appearance. Indeed, the term "honeycomb lung" has been used to describe severe interstitial restrictive lung disease.

Pleural diseases can also result in restriction of lung volume. The most striking example of this is what happens when air enters the pleural space — the space between the visceral pleura (the pleural membrane lining the lung) and the parietal pleura (the pleural membrane lining the inside of the chest wall). If air enters this space, the lung will collapse and this can restrict lung volume significantly. A simple spontaneous pneumothorax — air in the pleural space — is usually caused by the rupture of a small air space at the top of the lung. Five times more common among males than females, this problem seems most prevalent in young, tall, thin males and occurs in the right more often than the left lung.

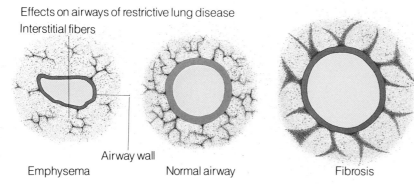

Effects on airways of restrictive lung disease

Interstitial fibers

Airway wall

Emphysema · Normal airway · Fibrosis

Restrictive disease has its own effects on the airways. In a patient with emphysema, the airways tend to collapse as radial traction is reduced by the disruption of surrounding fibers. In fibrosis the opposite occurs: fiber traction is increased, producing airways of increased diameter.

When the lung collapses, its volume is obviously reduced. As long as the leak of air does not continue, the air in the pleural space is gradually absorbed over days and weeks and the lung expands again. More complicated forms of pneumothorax can occur after injury to the chest. A puncture wound, for example, can cause a so-called open (sucking) pneumothorax. With each breath, more air from the outside is drawn into the pleural space, resulting in further collapse of the lung. Eventually the other lung becomes compressed and, if the air is not evacuated from the pleural space, this can be a threat to life.

If the lung is injured, but the chest wall entry site opens only during inspiration and closes like a flap during expiration, a tension pneumothorax can develop: with each breath, more and more air enters but does not leave the chest, resulting in a high, dangerous pressure on the heart and opposite lung. To treat a tension pneumothorax, a tube is inserted into the pleural space, and the air under pressure is evacuated.

Chest wall disease can cause hypoventilation, as mentioned earlier. Distortion of the bony thorax, respiratory muscle disease and obesity all restrict the volume of the lung, even though the lung itself is not diseased. All are disorders that result in a restrictive ventilatory defect. Patients with neuromuscular disease, chest wall disease and severe obesity have similar patterns of breathing — often rapid and shallow with reduced vital capacity. Sophisticated testing techniques demonstrate, however, that the lungs of such patients are usually normal and, unlike the lungs of patients suffering from pulmonary fibrosis or sarcoidosis, not stiff, or noncompliant.

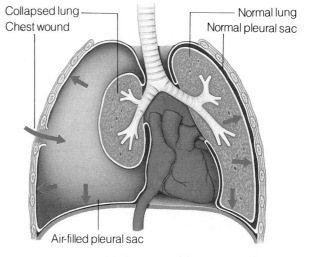

Collapsed lung
Chest wound

Normal lung
Normal pleural sac

Air-filled pleural sac

A chest wound is one cause of pneumothorax, or collapsed lung. With each intake of breath, air enters the pleural sac through the wound, causing the pleural sac to expand and the lung on that side to collapse. Although some, but less, air leaves the sac with each expiration, unless quickly treated, the lung continues to collapse as air builds up. The first priority is to cover the wound, to prevent more air from entering the chest until the patient can be treated and the lung reinflated.

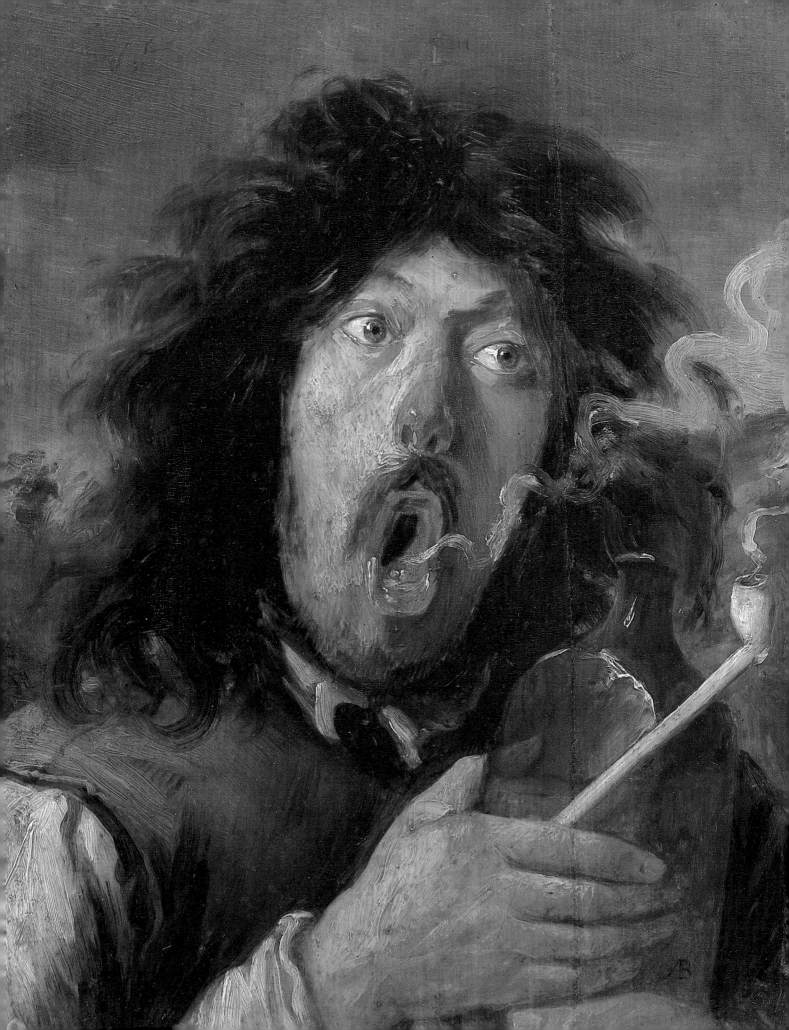

Chapter 5

Disorders of the Lungs

Since breathing is vital to a human being's survival, it is obvious that any disease of the respiratory system is potentially serious. Minor respiratory illnesses, such as colds and influenza, cause discomfort to millions and the loss of many work hours, while conditions such as emphysema and lung cancer are among the most common causes of death in the United States today.

Diseases of the respiratory system in which the cause is known and understood can be classified accordingly; for example, congenital, inhalational and infectious diseases can be grouped in this way. Airways disease and pulmonary vascular diseases are examples of conditions classified according to the parts of the body primarily involved in the disease process. Cancer of the lung is best classified according to the microscopic appearance of the cells. Some diseases, however, affect many different areas of the lung and their causes are unknown; for example, sarcoidosis, in which fleshy lesions appear in many parts of the body, including the lungs, and interstitial pulmonary fibrosis.

Congenital malformations result from abnormal development of parts of the body during fetal life. The development of the respiratory system can go wrong in a number of ways, and subsequent malformations of the chest wall and thoracic spine, the diaphragm, the trachea, the lungs themselves, the bronchi or the pulmonary blood vessels can all give rise to disease. For instance, pulmonary sequestrations and bronchogenic cysts may lead to pulmonary disease later in life. (The word "sequestered" means "hidden away.") Sometimes, as the lung develops, a portion grows that is not connected to the airways, blood supply or the tissue of the surrounding lung, and is thus hidden away without any communication with the outside world. The blood supply to this hidden section of lung often comes from the abdomen, outside the thorax. Eventually, pulmonary sequestrations tend to become infected and must be removed.

Cigarette smoking, once considered a sophisticated, sociable habit, has now indisputably been linked with respiratory diseases such as lung cancer, bronchitis and emphysema. The tobacco smoke so atmospherically shrouding the subject of Le Fumeur, *by Joos van Craesbeck (1605–62), contains many toxic compounds which assault and irritate the respiratory system.*

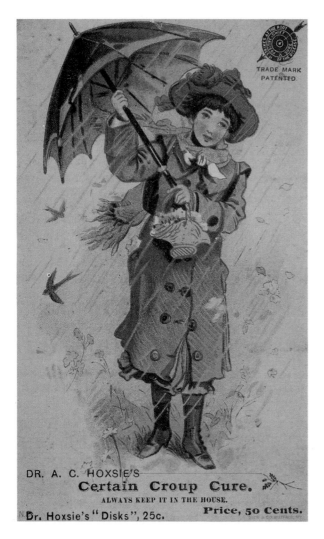

Croup, an illness generally suffered by young children, is a form of obstruction of the airways caused by acute inflammation of the laryngeal region. In young children the airways are extremely small and any swelling makes them narrower still, easily leading to breathing difficulties and the characteristic "croupy cough." Treatment aims to reduce inflammation and restore the free flow of air.

Bronchogenic cysts are congenital malformations that result from an abnormal budding or branching of the embryo's bronchial tree. A cyst, or empty cavity, within the lung or in the area of the heart and great vessels is formed and remains into adult life. The infection that ultimately arises must be treated with antibiotics and surgery.

Airways Disease

Pulmonary disease can also be brought about by obstructions of the trachea and bronchi. Obstruction of the upper airways — the trachea, larynx or vocal cords — can be the result of a variety of disorders, such as the external compression of the airways by tumors of the thyroid gland, or by tumors or polyps within the trachea or larynx. Patients with these conditions make noisy, high-pitched sounds as they breathe in. Paralysis of the vocal cords, injury to the neck, enlarged tonsils and "croup," or swelling of the laryngeal region, in children are yet more causes of airway obstruction.

The most dramatic cause of complete sudden upper airway obstruction is the inhalation of a foreign body, which may lodge in the larynx and totally obstruct airflow. Sometimes called a "café coronary," such obstruction often occurs during a meal, when a person inhales a piece of food such as steak or lobster; if not helped quickly, the person may die from asphyxiation. The best emergency treatment is the Heimlich maneuver — an upward thrust is delivered to the patient's abdomen to force air out of the lungs and clear the airway.

Asthma, chronic bronchitis and emphysema all obstruct airflow in different ways, as described in the previous chapter, but there is a considerable overlap of these disorders. A patient suffering from recurrent bronchospasm is diagnosed as having asthma, while a patient with a chronic mucus-producing cough as a consequence of repeated exposure to bronchial irritants, such as cigarette smoke, is said to have chronic bronchitis. In many patients, prolonged exposure to cigarette smoke results in increased mucus production, accompanied by increased susceptibility to infection, destructive and obstructive changes in the bronchial tubes and severe gas exchange problems. In the condition known as emphysema, gas exchange is reduced in dilated terminal airways and the

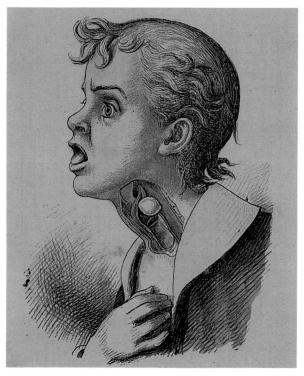

surrounding air space walls are destroyed. Chronic bronchitis, emphysema and asthma are all forms of chronic obstructive pulmonary disease (COPD) and features of each can coexist in the same patient.

By far the most common chronic lung disease, COPD is a serious public health problem. About 3.3 percent of the US population is estimated to have chronic bronchitis, and 0.66 to 0.97 percent emphysema. COPD is the fifth most common cause of death in the United States — in 1976, in the United States, 43,907 people died from chronic bronchitis or emphysema — and it is estimated that 4.8 billion dollars a year is spent on treatment and hospital care for those suffering from the condition.

Smoking is the single most important reason for chronic bronchitis and emphysema. COPD is uncommon in nonsmokers, and ex-cigarette smokers have lower death rates from COPD than do continuing smokers. While pollution or occupational hazards are less important than smoking as an agent of COPD, in combination with smoking they can act to worsen the condition. Even in

Section through cartilage hoop   Gland ducts

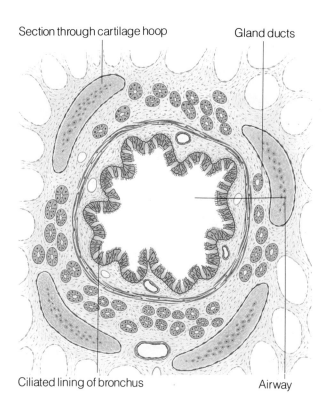

Ciliated lining of bronchus   Airway

In its normal state a bronchus (left) has an unobstructed airway. If disease is present, the bronchus may become narrowed, either because the surrounding ring of muscle tightens and constricts it or because it is obstructed by excessive mucus, which the cilia cannot clear.

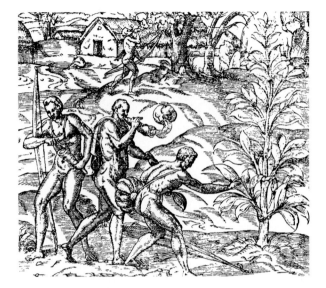

Tobacco was introduced into Europe in the 1560s by Christopher Columbus who, when he landed in America, found natives using the material. The first known printed illustration of smoking, this sixteenth-century drawing depicts natives gathering, rolling and smoking leaves of the tobacco plant.

smokers without overt symptoms of chronic obstructive pulmonary disease, lung function tests often reveal abnormalities. In the 1980s, COPD is three or four times more common in men than women, but as the smoking habits of women change, this difference may not be as great in the future. Since the 1960s, far more men than women have given up smoking.

A family history of chronic bronchitis or emphysema may predispose a patient to these diseases. There is a rare, familial type of emphysema caused by an inherited deficiency of alpha-l-antitrypsin, a chemical that prevents the action of enzymes which can break down lung tissue. In those who inherit the abnormal gene causing this condition, emphysema often starts in their third or fourth decade — even in nonsmokers. Less than one percent of those with emphysema belong in this category, however.

Patients with COPD may have a history of suffering chronic cough and producing large amounts of sputum; they may have frequent respiratory infections over the years, accompanied by the production of thick sputum and by wheezing. Shortness of breath on exertion may not be as noticeable in the early stages but will worsen and eventually limit activity. Late in the disease, patients may experience low levels of oxygen in the blood, sleep disturbances, headaches, hypercorbia (an abnormally high level of carbon dioxide in the blood), pulmonary hypertension and right-sided heart failure, and even personality changes.

Pink Puffers and Blue Bloaters

There are two types of COPD patient. Those with predominant emphysema are referred to as "pink puffers" because their oxygen levels are usually satisfactory, so they remain "pink," and because they develop a pursed-lipped style of breathing, taking rapid, shallow, puffing breaths. "Blue bloaters," patients with predominant chronic bronchitis, are so called because their low oxygen levels give them a blue look and because they suffer heart failure and swell with fluid. The low oxygen levels occur because the mucus irregularly obstructs the airways which continue to be perfused with blood.

The most important therapy for patients with

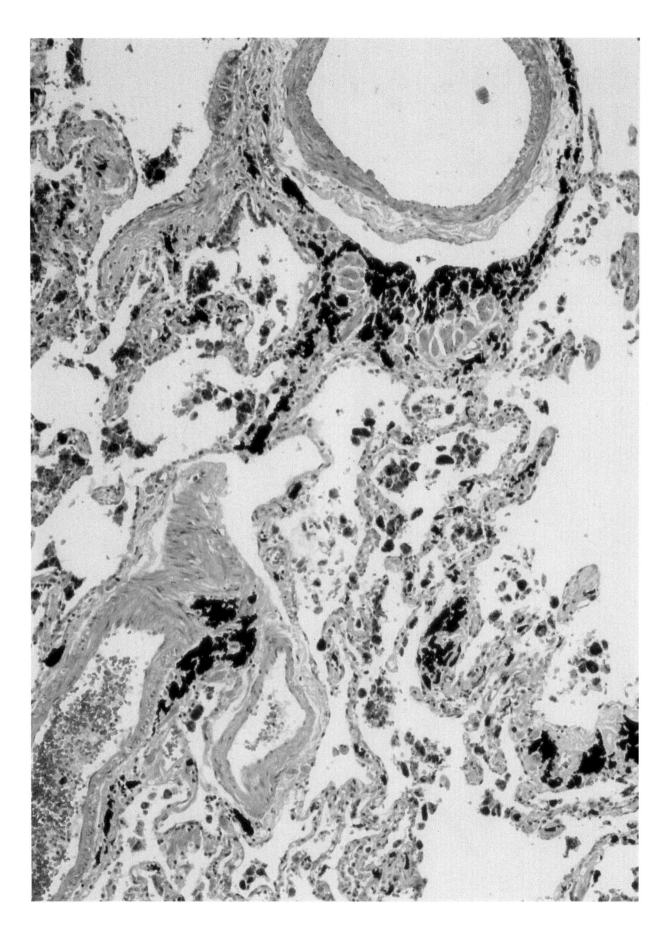

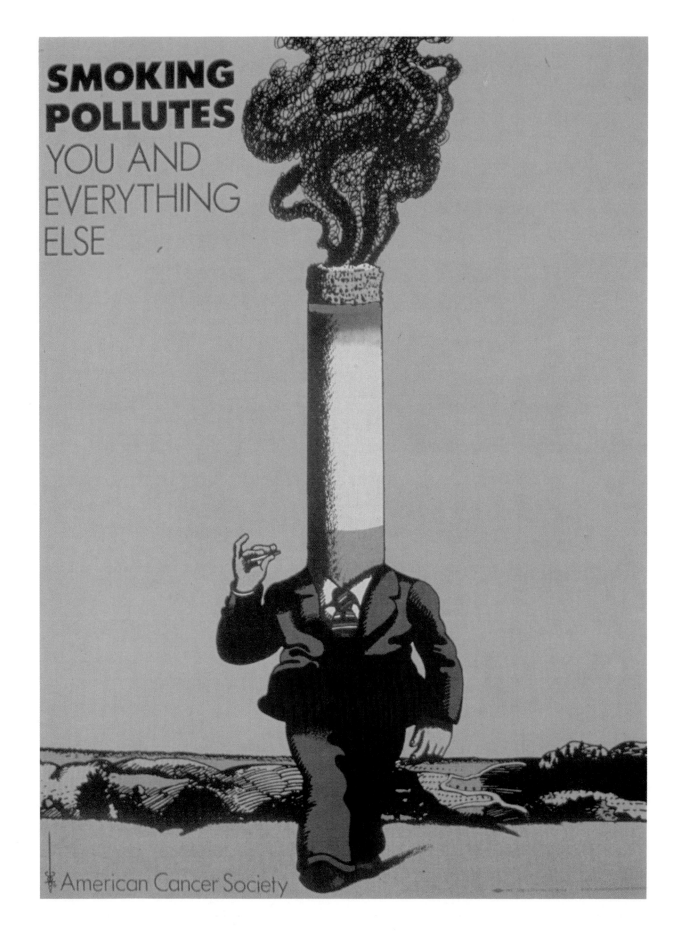

Drawing attention to the dangers of "secondhand smoke" is an important part of the antismoking campaign. Researchers estimate that two-thirds of the smoke from a burning cigarette goes into the environment

Asthma attacks, and the allergic reaction known as hay fever, can have many triggers, one of which is the pollen of a variety of plants. A dramatic solution to the problem has been found by this group of people.

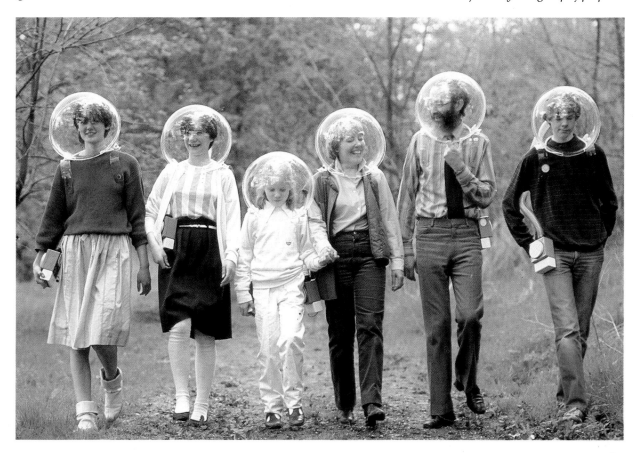

chronic bronchitis and emphysema is to stop cigarette smoking. Hypnotism, behavior modification techniques, nicotine gum and many other aids are tried by smokers, with variable success. If patients do stop smoking, however, symptoms decrease, and they are less likely to suffer further deterioration of lung function.

Giving up smoking is particularly important — and rewarding — for patients with early mild signs of COPD revealed by lung function testing. Once these patients stop smoking, the lungs do not deteriorate further and COPD can be prevented.

Patients with established COPD can be helped by medications which relax the bronchial tubes (bronchodilators), antibiotics to treat bacterial infection, and corticosteriod drugs to reduce the inflammation. Physical exercise programs, breathing exercises and portable supplemental oxygen are all important treatments in the late stages of COPD.

Approximately 3 percent of the population of the United States has asthma. In asthma, the airways are contracted by muscle reaction and further obstructed by an increase in mucus secretion and swelling of wall tissues. All of this leaves little room for air to be expired, so causing the characteristic wheezing sounds made by asthmatics. Other characteristic symptoms include spells of shortness of breath and, in some patients, coughing. Asthma often begins in childhood and in 75 percent of cases becomes less severe in adolescence, although about 25 percent of asthmatics do continue to suffer symptoms in adult life.

The Triggers of Asthma

Most cases of asthma in children and adolescents are associated with an allergic reaction of a particularly sensitive bronchial tree to pollen, certain foods, house mites, dusts and animal danders — all of which may trigger attacks. Such agents, or allergens, react with antibodies and

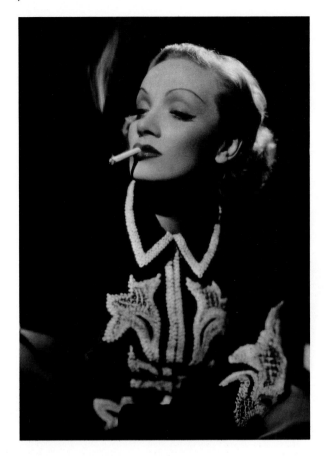

induce the release of potent, naturally occurring chemicals. These make the muscles in the walls of the bronchial tubes contract, thus bringing about respiratory difficulties.

Asthma can also be triggered by infections, exercise, inhalation of cold air, certain medications, especially aspirin, and, in many people, by psychological or emotional factors. If a person over the age of thirty-five develops asthma, it rarely has a predominantly allergic cause and may often be difficult to distinguish from chronic bronchitis.

An important part of asthma therapy is to identify and, where possible, avoid any triggers or precipitating factors. Medications to relax the bronchial tubes and control allergic symptoms are often helpful, and physical exercise and normal activity should be encouraged.

Bronchiectasis and cystic fibrosis are other important airway diseases. Bronchiectasis means "stretched bronchi"; these enlarged bronchial tubes drain off the mucus secretions ineffectively and, therefore, are particularly susceptible to recurrent infections. In Kartagener's syndrome, a congenital disease in which the heart is on the right instead of the left side of the chest, bronchiectasis as well as sinus problems occur. Such patients have a defect in the movement of cilia, the hairlike structures lining the respiratory cells that normally beat to clear secretions out of the bronchial tubes. In males with this condition, the tails on sperm cells are also immobile, and these men are usually infertile. Bronchiectasis and obstructive lung disease are also part of cystic fibrosis, an inherited disease which also affects the pancreas and causes thick bronchial secretions to be produced.

Tumors of the Lung

One of the most common and serious of all lung diseases, lung cancer has been on the increase since the turn of the twentieth century: it is estimated that in the 1980s more than 130,000 people in the United States die from it each year. The most common tumor of the lung — and the disease usually referred to as lung cancer, or bronchogenic carcinoma — is a cancer arising from a bronchus.

Lung cancer is more common in men than women; in 1960 about 85 percent of cases were men, 15 percent women. The number of women suffering from lung cancer is on the increase, however, and is strongly linked to the increase in smoking by women in recent decades — in the 1930s and 1940s cigarette smoking became a glamorous thing for women to do. If the trend continues, lung cancer may soon equal or surpass breast cancer as the number one cancer killer in women.

The link between smoking and lung cancer is beyond doubt. About one in ten heavy smokers (people who smoke twenty cigarettes or more each day) eventually suffers lung cancer, and the risk of dying from the disease is as much as eighteen times greater in smokers than nonsmokers. Air pollution and living and working in an urban environment may add to the risk of developing lung cancer, but these factors are small when compared to the effects of smoking. Working in mines with radioactive ores, or exposure to asbestos, especially

The highest incidence of lung cancer is in people between the ages of 55 and 75. This X ray of the front of the chest of a cancer patient shows established lesions of bronchial carcinoma in the left lung.

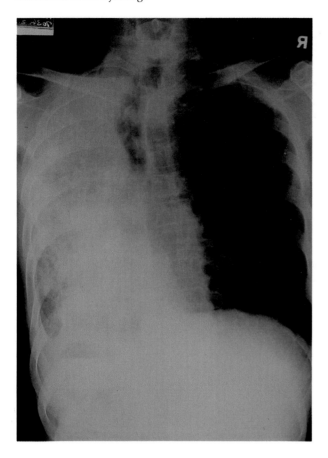

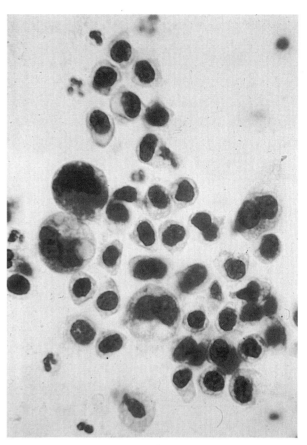

Carcinoma of the bronchial gland cells, adenocarcinoma, is here magnified many hundreds of times. Provided that it has not spread outside the lungs, this type of cancer can sometimes be removed by surgery.

in combination with cigarette smoking, are more significant risk factors.

There are four types of cancer of the bronchus, or bronchogenic carcinoma. The most common is squamous cell carcinoma, a malignant growth in the skinlike cells lining the bronchial tube. The next most common, and the type of tumor which most often spreads to other parts of the body, is oat cell carcinoma, with small, round, immature cells. The third type is adenocarcinoma which arises from bronchial glandular cells (adeno means gland), and the fourth is large cell cancer.

Cancer of the lung has various effects on the respiratory system. It may obstruct a bronchus, which can cause pneumonia or collapse of the lung beyond it. Fluid may collect in the pleural space due to the presence of tumor, or important organs in the chest, such as major blood vessels and nerves controlling the diaphragm and vocal cords, may be compressed or invaded.

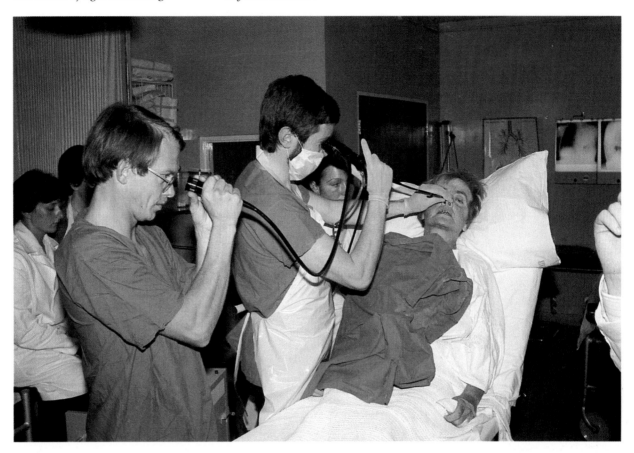

Coughing is one early symptom of lung cancer (and of many other conditions); there may be spitting of blood, and patients often lose weight. Sometimes the first sign is in an area outside the chest, such as an enlarged lymph node in the neck or even a distant (metastatic) spread of the cancer to the bones, liver or brain. In some cases there are no symptoms at all until a shadow is noticed on a routine chest X ray; small round tumors, or "coin lesions," are common early signs found in this way.

Another way of examining the bronchial tubes is with the aid of a bronchoscope. This is a flexible instrument with a lens and light source which is inserted through the nose or mouth, down the throat and into the bronchial tubes; the physician can then see what, if anything, is in the bronchus. Sometimes exploratory surgery is necessary for complete diagnosis.

Lung cancer is treated by surgery, radiation therapy or chemotherapy. For squamous cell cancers and adenocarcinomas, surgery, if possible, is the best therapy. Oat cell cancers are best treated with chemotherapy and radiation therapy because they are always widespread when diagnosed. Unfortunately, the survival rate for lung cancer patients remains low, but better treatments are constantly being tested and researched. About one percent of lung cancer patients have alveolar cell carcinoma, tumors that originate in the cells lining the alveoli. This type of cancer does not seem to be directly related to cigarette smoking.

Some lung tumors, such as bronchial carcinoid tumor, are benign. Although not as dangerous as malignant lung cancers, benign tumors can still cause bronchial obstruction, pneumonia, bleeding and chronic cough, and surgical removal is the best treatment. One type of cancer, a tumor of the pleura — the lining of the lungs — is strongly linked to exposure to asbestos. The exposure may be brief and the tumor may develop thirty to fifty years

Over a hundred cold-causing viruses have so far been identified; one type is illustrated here by a computer graphics technique. Cold viruses are spread in droplets of moisture expelled while coughing or sneezing.

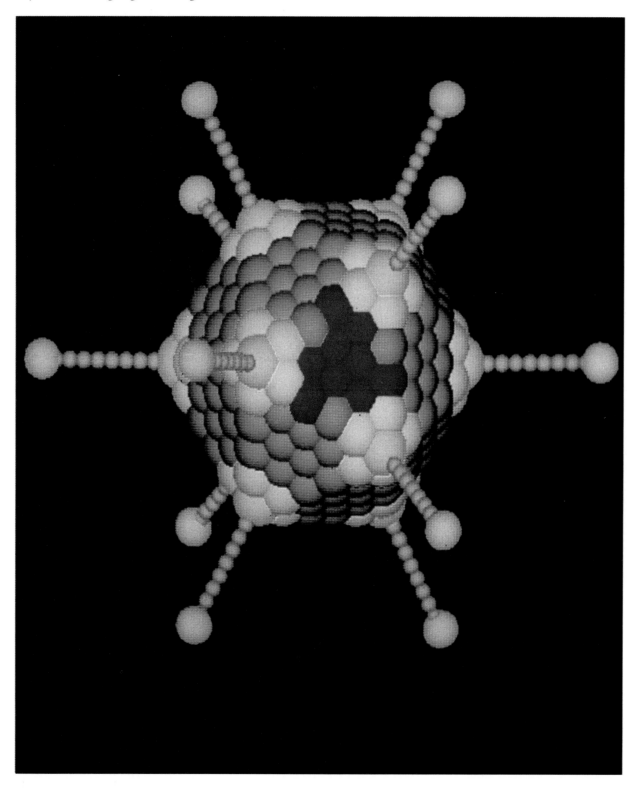

The virus causing Asian flu is here
magnified many thousands of times.
Vaccination against influenza is now
available, using vaccine made from
the major viral strains present in
any year.

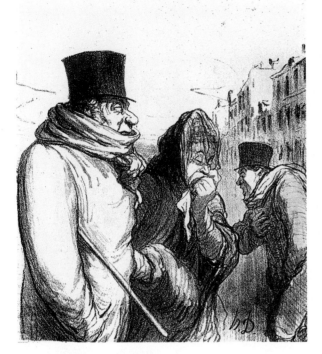

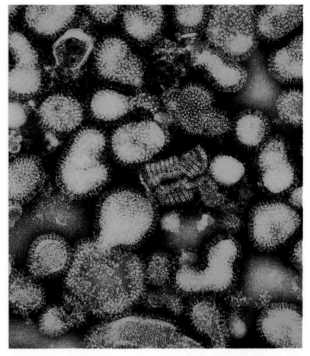

Influenza, too, is caused by virus.
Every decade or so a new virus
strain appears to which people have
no immunity, and an epidemic can
ensue. The 1918 flu virus spread
worldwide and caused twenty
million deaths. This illustration by
French painter and satirist Honoré
Daumier (1808–79) shows the plight
of unhappy Parisians in the throes of
an earlier epidemic.

later. A patient suffering from this tumor, malignant mesothelioma, may complain of chest pain or shortness of breath, but in many cases, there are simply vague complaints of fatigue. Currently there is no effective treatment for this rare type of tumor.

Respiratory infections are common causes of illness in both previously healthy individuals and in patients with a more serious underlying condition. Colds and influenza are experienced by almost everyone at some time; but, more seriously, bacteria, viruses, tuberculosis, fungi and protozoal organisms can infect the lungs and cause pneumonia. Broadly an inflammation of the lungs, pneumonia causes the alveoli to fill with mucus and fluid, so impairing gas exchange and, as a result, the functioning of the whole body. There are three main causes of acute pneumonia: bacteria, viruses and mycoplasmas.

Bacterial pneumonia is most often caused by the bacteria *Streptococcus pneumoniae*, or the *pneumococcus*, although many other types of bacteria can also be responsible. Bacteria are usually inhaled and, once they reach the alveoli, cause inflammation and the accumulation of fluid and white blood cells. When the alveoli become filled in this way, that

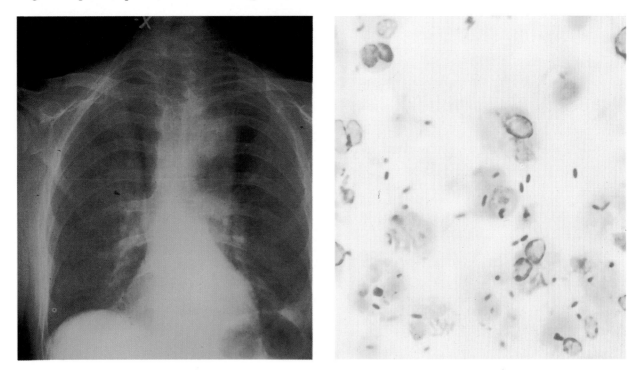

area of the lung becomes solid, or consolidated, and shows up as such on a chest X ray. Patients usually suffer from fever, a sputum-producing cough, shaking, chills and chest pain; the sputum may occasionally be streaked with blood. If a significant amount of lung tissue is affected, the intake of oxygen and gas exchange are impaired; in severe cases this can lead to respiratory failure and death.

Penicillin is the most effective antibiotic against pneumococcal pneumonia, but other antibiotics are also used, since many of the organisms that cause pneumonia are resistant to penicillin.

Pneumonia due to a different type of bacteria was responsible for a well-known outbreak of illness at an American Legion convention in Philadelphia in 1976. Now called Legionnaire's disease, this type of pneumonia can be quite severe, but it is effectively treated by antibiotics. It most often occurs after exposure to soil or stagnant water where the bacterial organism naturally occurs, and outbreaks are frequently tied to recent excavation or construction work, or to contaminated water or air conditioning systems.

As many as half of all pneumonia cases are caused by viruses; this type can be mild or, in some cases, severe and life threatening. Symptoms are flulike, with fever, aching joints and muscles, headache, watering eyes and nasal congestion, cough and sore throat. There is no specific therapy for most viral infections, but supportive treatment with aspirin or other fever-reducing drugs, combined with plenty of fluids and rest, seems to be helpful.

The third type, mycoplasma pneumonia, is caused by an organism that resembles a virus in some ways and a bacterium in others. Sometimes known as "atypical pneumonia," mycoplasma is generally a mild illness in young adults, with its most prominent symptom being a dry, hacking cough. A chest X ray usually shows patchy shadows on the lung, rather than one solid area. The same antibiotic as that used against Legionnaire's disease, erythromycin, is also helpful in treating mycoplasma infection.

Patients suffering from diseases that impair the body's ability to fight off infection can develop unusual pneumonias. For example, patients with kidney transplants or certain types of cancer have poor defense systems, as do premature or malnourished infants. In the condition commonly

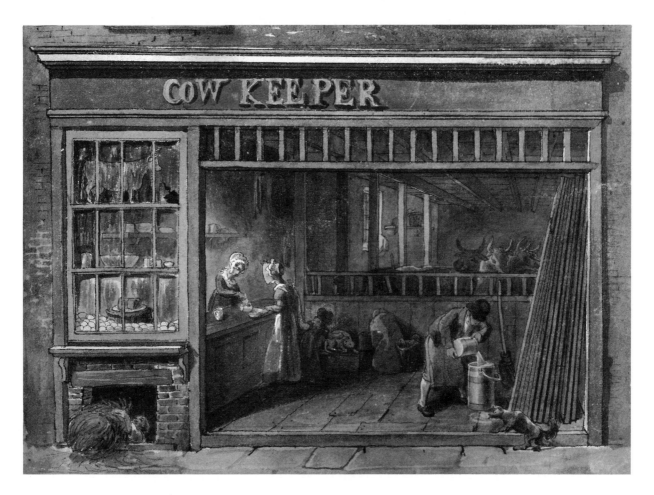

known as AIDS (acquired immuno-deficiency syndrome) — suffered primarily by homosexuals — a defect in the immune system is acquired due to a viral infection. Such patients commonly contract pneumonia, which can progress rapidly and, if untreated, is almost always fatal; even with appropriate treatment, pneumonia in an AIDS patient is associated with high mortality.

Tuberculosis, an infectious disease which usually begins in the lungs, was once one of the leading causes of death worldwide. In 1900, in the United States, there were 100 deaths per 100,000 of the population, and 200 new cases per 100,000 were reported every year around this time. During this "pre-antibiotic era" — the period before the introduction of safe, effective, antituberculosis therapy — TB patients were sent to sanitariums where it was thought that rest and fresh air would help cure the disease. Many of the physicians working in these sanitariums also suffered from tuberculosis.

The main benefit of sending patients to the "magic mountain," as Thomas Mann called the tuberculosis sanitarium in his novel of that name, was to isolate them and prevent them from spreading the disease. However, some patients did improve as their own immune systems controlled the disease.

As living conditions and public hygiene improved during the early years of the twentieth century, the incidence and mortality rate of tuberculosis decreased, even before the introduction of antituberculosis therapy. Young people exposed to tuberculosis often did not develop the disease to any significant extent and, instead, developed enhanced immunity.

Antituberculosis therapy was introduced in the 1950s; by 1976, the mortality rate in the United States had fallen to 1.4 per 100,000 people. The disease still has a high incidence, however, in the underdeveloped countries of the world and in low socioeconomic groups in industrialized countries.

Tuberculosis is associated with poverty and overcrowded, poorly ventilated living conditions, and also with poor nutrition, alcoholism, underlying complaints such as diabetes, Hodgkin's disease or other malignancies, and their treatment. Lung diseases, with the exception of silicosis, have not so far been linked with an increased incidence of tuberculosis.

Infection with the bovine type of TB bacillus via milk, once the cause of at least some cases, is now rare. It has been virtually eliminated by the pasteurization of milk and regular testing of dairy cattle.

Once one of the major causes of death in the United States, tuberculosis is now treatable and far less common. There is no longer any need for the isolation of patients seen in this TB ward of 1890.

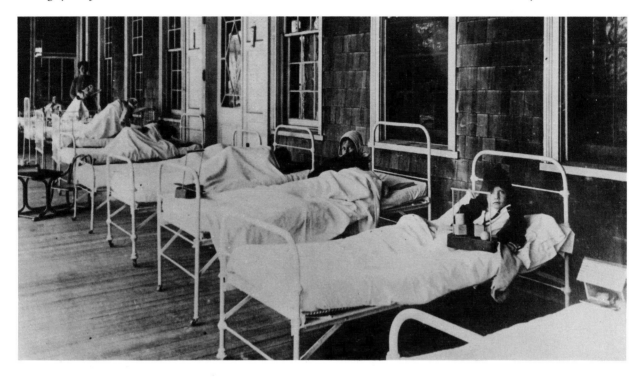

The cause of tuberculosis is the organism *Mycobacterium tuberculosis*. If a person with the disease coughs or sneezes, droplets containing organisms are discharged into the air and can be inhaled by someone in close personal contact. Once inhaled, the tubercle bacilli become implanted in the alveoli of the lung and usually produce a reaction similar to any acute pneumonia. Within a day or two, organisms are carried to all parts of the body. Three to ten weeks later, there is a characteristic inflammatory reaction consisting of an aggregation of white blood cells (lymphocytes, histiocytes, giant cells) and some fibrous tissue — a granuloma. In individuals with normal resistance, the tubercle bacilli are killed or walled in by this process; the granuloma eventually scars down and becomes calcified like bone.

Tubercle bacilli also travel through the lymphatic channels to the lymph nodes, which may become enlarged. The combination of a granulomatous lesion in the lung and enlarged lymph nodes draining that region of the lung is termed the primary infection. This initial focus of infection can occur anywhere in the lung, but reactivation of tuberculosis is characteristically in the upper lobes.

Sometimes the primary infection results in serious disease of the lung or spreads through the bloodstream to cause disease throughout the body. In the latter case, there are multiple small areas of infection in the lungs which are said to resemble millet seeds; hence this type of TB is known as miliary tuberculosis. Potentially serious, it is often associated with meningitis due to tuberculosis.

Reactivated TB
The number of organisms entering the bloodstream is generally small and they may be killed or may survive in a dormant state. Dormant organisms may reactivate many years after the primary infection has healed and this is the prime cause of TB today. Many years earlier, a person may have breathed in TB bacteria which were successfully resisted and walled in by granuloma. If that person's resistance is weakened, for one reason or another, the bacteria may become active again and start to do damage.

Reactivation of tuberculosis in the lungs tends to produce disease in the upper lobes where, in a person standing upright, oxygen tension is slightly higher than in the lower lobes. The tubercle bacilli

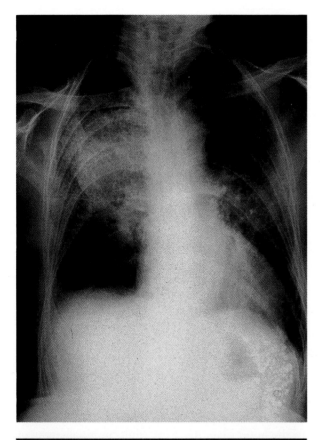

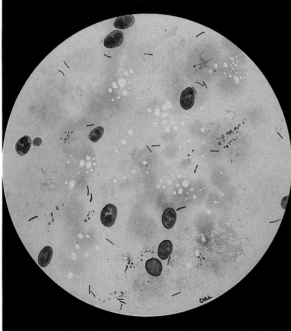

need oxygen to multiply and, therefore, have a better chance in the upper zones. Reactivated tuberculosis often causes a cavity, or hole, to form in the upper lobe of the lung; cheesy, or caseous, material containing many tubercle bacilli can then spill into the bronchial tree and spread or be coughed up. If the disease is not treated, it causes scarring and recurrent lung destruction.

The onset of tuberculosis is often slow and vague and, therefore, difficult to diagnose. Patients may notice fatigue and loss of appetite or weight loss; coughing, blood spitting, fevers and night sweats may be other symptoms.

One way of diagnosing TB is by a skin test in which protein derivatives of the tubercle bacilli are injected into the skin. If the subject develops a raised red spot on the skin as a reaction to this injection, he or she may have tuberculosis and should have a chest X ray. If the chest X ray is abnormal in an upper lung lobe there is good reason to suspect tuberculosis, and the patient's sputum should be tested for tubercle bacilli.

Nowadays the disease can be easily and effectively treated with antituberculosis antibiotics. There is rarely a need for patients to be hospitalized, and most can continue to lead a normal life during treatment. Once a case of tuberculosis has been confirmed, the patient's family and other close contacts should be tested for the disease, since treatment with antibiotics can protect them from contracting TB.

Infection with fungi, or molds, can occur in the lung and may resemble TB on a chest X ray. Two such fungal diseases occurring in the United States are histoplasmosis and coccidioidomycosis.

Histoplasmosis is common in the Mississippi and Ohio river valleys but also occurs throughout the rest of the world. It is caused by infection by the fungus *Histoplasma capsulatum*, and dusts containing the spores of this mold are often found in caves, basements or chicken coops. The primary infection is usually a mild, flulike illness, or it may even be without symptoms: old calcified scars due to unnoticed infections are frequently discovered on X rays of people from the Ohio river valley area. However, as in tuberculosis, infection may spread throughout the body or form a cavity in the lungs.

Coccidioidomycosis is a similar disease caused by

Robert Koch

Waging War on Tuberculosis

"I have undertaken my investigations in the interests of public health and I hope the greatest benefits will accrue therefrom." So wrote Robert Koch, one of the greatest bacteriologists of all time, when he embarked upon his lifelong quest — the control of tuberculosis.

The third son of Lutheran parents, Koch was born in Germany in 1843. An intelligent child, he dreamed of being an explorer and seeing the world. He studied medicine at a time when scientists all over Europe were fiercely debating Louis Pasteur's bacteriological work on fermentation. Robert Koch graduated from the University of Göttingen in 1866, married the following year and, after several unsettled years, was appointed District Medical Officer at Wollstein. In this lakeside town, Koch and his family spent eight happy years.

A tireless, methodical worker, Koch discovered, during his time at Wollstein, the bacteria responsible for causing anthrax in cattle. The following year he laid down guidelines for the fixing, staining and microphotographic recording of bacteria and in 1878 published what became known as "Koch's Postulates." These were rules for a thoroughly satisfactory proof for correctly identifying the causative agent of a disease.

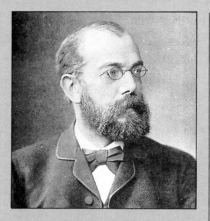

After he was appointed government advisor with the Department of Health in Berlin in 1880, one member of his team remarked: "Almost daily new miracles of bacteriology displayed themselves before our astonished eyes."

It was alone, and in secret, however, that Koch started his work on tuberculosis. It took him six months to prove what he already believed: that TB was chronically infectious. On March 24, 1882, Koch announced to the Physiological Society of Berlin that he had positively identified the bacillus that caused one of the worst diseases to afflict mankind. Only a man of Koch's determination could have isolated this bacillus — so small and difficult to find. With its waxy coat it was also difficult to stain, and its slow growth and nutritional requirements made it hard to culture.

Koch was acclaimed for his work and his genius was much in demand. He traveled to Egypt and India and there identified the causative agent of amoebic dysentery and the cholera bacillus. Back in Berlin, he began his search for a remedy for TB. In 1890, he announced that he had "at last hit upon a substance with the power of preventing the growth of the tubercle bacillus." Hopes were high, and for a while Koch was honored and congratulated, as doctors and patients flocked to Berlin to discover more about this miraculous new cure for tuberculosis.

But doubts soon arose about the efficacy of the new substance "tuberculin," and professional skepticism spread. His reputation on the wane, Koch traveled abroad for a while, returning to Berlin to work when the fuss had died down.

As well as investigating other diseases, such as bubonic plague and sleeping sickness, Koch continued his work on TB control, supervising production and clinical trials of new tuberculins. In 1905, he received the Nobel Prize for his work on the tubercle bacillus — work that has had far-reaching effects on all of medical science. Five years later, Koch suffered a severe attack of angina from which he failed to come round. He died peacefully in his chair at the Baden-Baden sanitarium.

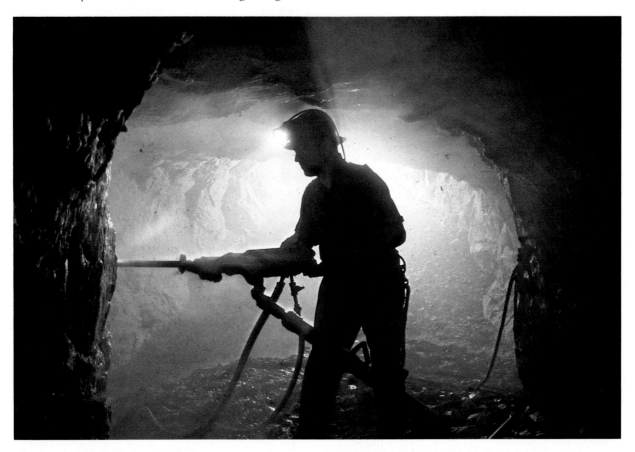

fungi spores which float in clouds of desert dust. It occurs in the southwestern desert areas of the United States in southern California, Arizona, Texas, Nevada, New Mexico and Utah. Symptoms of the primary infection are again flulike, although many infected people show no symptoms at all. If the disease spreads through the body, it can be serious and requires drug treatment and sometimes hospitalization. People traveling — even briefly — to the Southwest, as well as locals, are at risk, and details of recent journeys can help to diagnose this often puzzling illness.

Inhalational Lung Disease

In today's industrialized society there is more than we think in the air we breathe, and breathing in dusts and vapors found in the environment in which we live or work can be the cause of serious inhalational lung disease. Industrial, or occupational, lung disease is another term for the

problems that result from the long-term inhalation of dusts found in mines or other workplaces. Organic dust exposure, the inhalation of dusts from plant and animal sources, can also cause lung disease due to the allergic-type reactions they can produce in the lungs. Air pollution, too, can worsen existing lung disease, such as chronic bronchitis, while exposure to toxic gases can result in acute and chronic lung injury. Some dusts and gases can cause or aggravate asthma.

The inhalation of inorganic dusts is a serious problem in mining and other industries. The term pneumoconiosis describes disease caused by dust retained in the lung, while silicosis is a type of pneumoconiosis resulting from inhalation of dusts containing free crystalline silica. Free silica is produced in all types of mining in which ore is extracted from quartz-containing rock; there is also danger of silica exposure in ceramics manufacture, granite cutting and polishing, and coal mining.

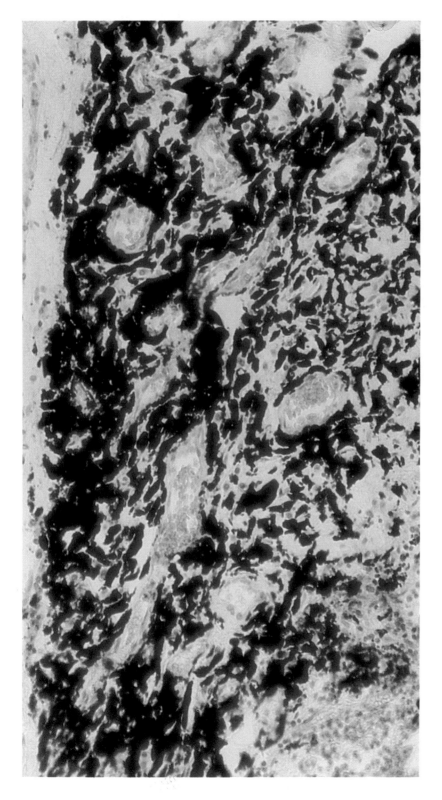

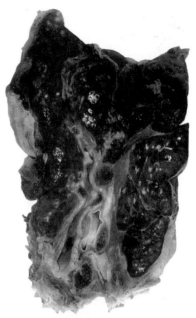

Inhalation of certain dusts and particles can cause diseases affecting the connective tissue of the lungs. In silicosis, tissues react to inhaled particles of silica. Nodules form around the particles, aggregate and start to distort and obstruct the airways, (above). Inhalation of coal dust causes coal worker's pneumoconiosis. The dust settles in the alveoli and bronchioles (left) and can cause scarring and lung damage.

*Particles of silica, the cause of the
inhalational lung disease silicosis,
are a hazard in industries such as
quarrying, mining and tunneling, or
in any process where sand is used as
an abrasive.*

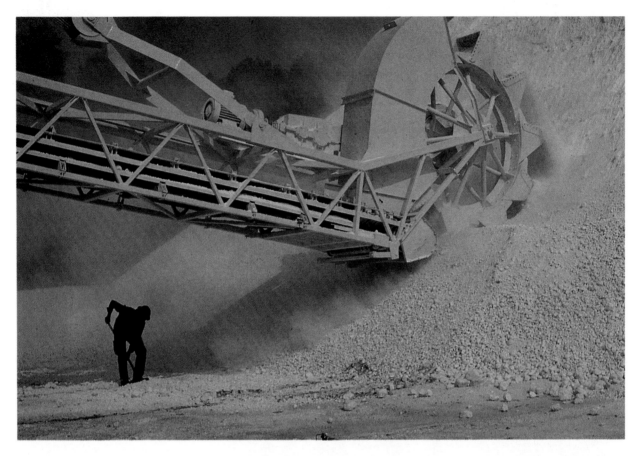

Construction workers, too, may be at risk, since silica is present in building materials (sandstone) and is used as an abrasive agent for sandblasting and in abrasive paper.

After at least five years exposure to silica dust the inhaled dust causes scarring in the lungs. After longer or excessive exposure, these scarred areas may enlarge and combine, resulting in the more serious form of the pneumoconiosis-type diseases, progressive massive fibrosis. The symptoms of this disease are variable, but it may cause severe shortness of breath, coughing and the production of black-stained sputum. Many patients, though, do not suffer serious disability.

Silicosis may be complicated by tuberculosis, and workers who smoke may also suffer from chronic obstructive pulmonary disease (COPD). Once silicosis is established, there is no good treatment, but efforts can be made toward its prevention. The National Institute of Occupational Safety and Health (NIOSH) is involved in setting up preventive measures in mining and other industries. Where proper ventilation and clearing of dust is not possible, workers may be advised to wear special masks and respirators: sandblasters in particular should wear masks with a supply of pressurized fresh air. All such employees should have pulmonary function tests to screen them for lung disease.

Coal workers' pneumoconiosis — also known as "black lung disease" — is caused by an accumulation of coal dust in the lungs. Exposure to silica in coal mining was thought to be the culprit in black lung disease, but it is now known that coal dust itself can be the cause.

Miners who show signs of the disease on chest X rays, but do not show serious abnormalities on pulmonary function testing, are said to have simple coal workers' pneumoconiosis. In complicated coal workers' pneumoconiosis, or progressive massive fibrosis, there is always a lowering of breathing

Asbestosis is caused by inhaled asbestos fibers, here visible as long bodies in lung tissue. The fibers lodge in the airways, eventually causing thickening and fibrosis of tissue surrounding air spaces.

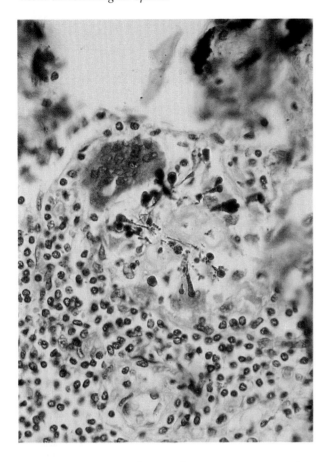

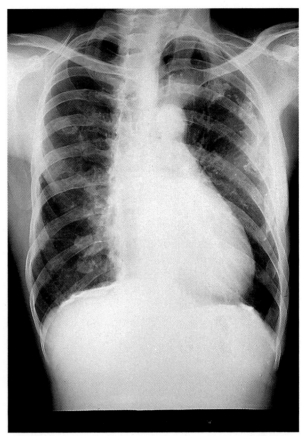

capacity. A miner who smokes cigarettes may also have chronic bronchitis and airflow obstruction.

The Risks of Asbestos

Asbestos, an important fire-proofing and insulating agent, has been linked with several different types of respiratory disease, including asbestosis, a chronic scarring of the lung similar to other pneumoconioses. In asbestosis, actual asbestos fibers may be seen on an X ray of the scarred lung. Asbestos can also cause benign pleural disease but, as mentioned previously, is linked with malignant mesothelioma — tumor of the pleura, the lining of the lungs. Smokers who have been exposed to asbestos have a much higher incidence of lung cancer: their risk is ninety times greater than that of normal nonsmokers and five to ten times greater than of smokers without asbestos exposure.

Although heavy exposure is most usual in mining and construction work, asbestos is found in

Pleural plaques, visible on X ray, can be one result of asbestosis. These raised lesions contain asbestos fibers and occur on the parietal pleura, the outer lining of the lung, over the area of the lower ribs and diaphragm.

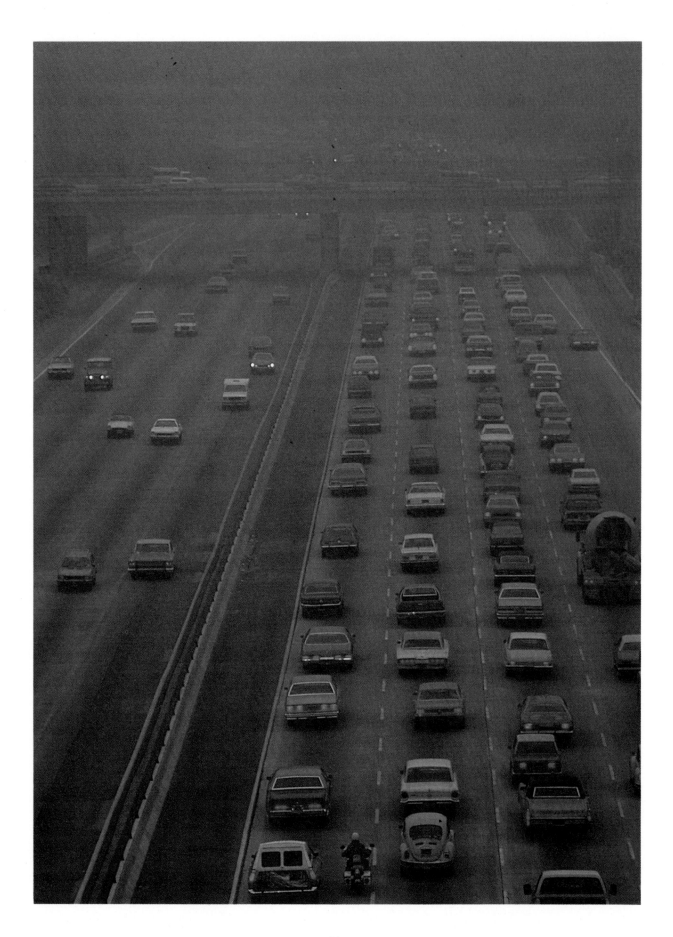

The millions of automobiles on our
roads are pouring tons of harmful
substances, such as carbon monoxide
and hydrocarbons, into the air every
year and are one of the most serious
sources of air pollution.

A Tokyo policeman takes oxygen
therapy following a shift on traffic
duty. There are now strict guidelines
on the length of time such personnel
may be exposed to the high level of
pollution caused by traffic.

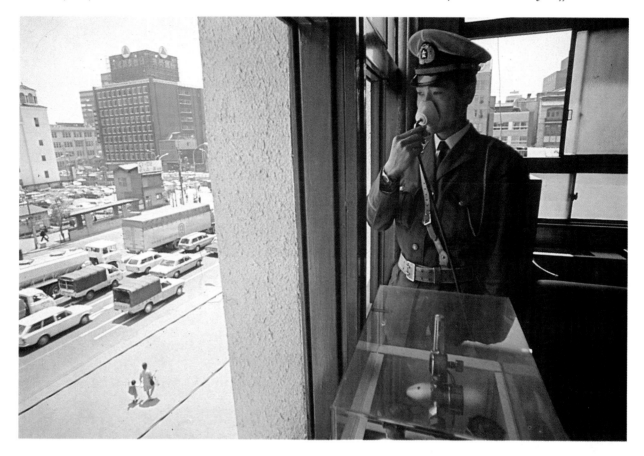

so many products that incidental exposure may be common. Brake pads in cars, insulation in homes and schools, roofing and floor tiles, plumbing and pipe insulation, and other household products may all contain asbestos.

Only prolonged, intense exposure produces the scarring of asbestosis, but malignant mesothelioma can occur after brief exposure and has often been reported in the wives of asbestos workers whose exposure came from laundering their husbands' dusty clothes. Efforts to control both the use of asbestos and exposure to it are important preventive measures.

Exposure to other organic dusts and certain metals can also cause lung disease. For example, the metal iron oxide, inhaled by arc welders; cadmium, which may be inhaled in the fumes produced by smelting ores; beryllium, used in the aerospace industry and in the manufacture of fluorescent light bulbs; tungsten, nickel and many

others. Toxic gases, too, are the source of problems. Ammonia fumes can produce pulmonary edema (fluid in the lungs) within a few hours of exposure, while heavier exposure may cause chronic bronchitis and other abnormalities revealed by X ray. Exposure to oxides of nitrogen can result in lung disease in arc welders, in industrial workers exposed to nitric acid and in workers exposed to fermenting corn in a closed silo (silo filler's disease).

Hazards in the Air

Air pollution affects everyone in the country indiscriminately. The American Lung Association estimates that the damage pollution causes to health, property, materials and vegetation costs the country some 20 billion dollars a year. Air is polluted primarily by carbon monoxide and hydrocarbons (mostly from automobiles), sulfur oxides, (from burning coal and fuel oil), particulate matter (particles of solid or liquid matter emanating

Industrial processes, giving out both particles and gases, are another source of pollution. Particularly harmful to those already suffering respiratory disease, pollution may also lower the defenses of the healthy.

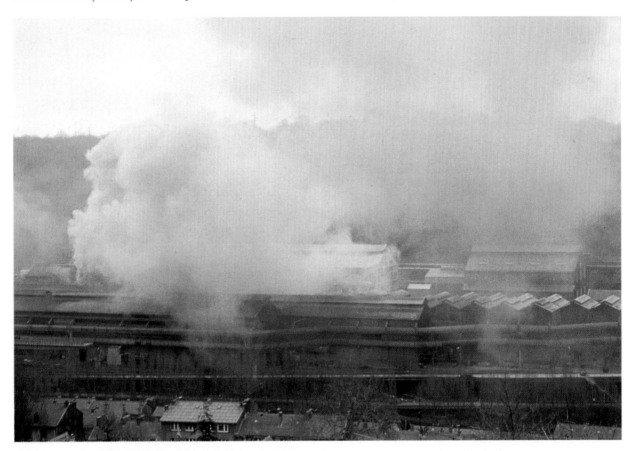

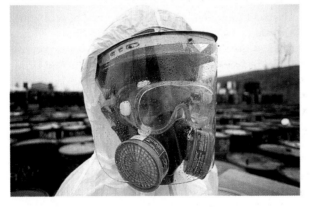

In the United States, it is estimated that 60,000 workers each year contract work-related respiratory disease. Those at risk should take all possible precautions and should be supplied with protective equipment if necessary.

from almost every industrial process), nitrogen oxides (from automobiles and steam power plants) and photochemical oxidants — the smog formed by substances such as ozone, produced by the action of sunlight on hydrocarbons and nitrogen oxides.

Air containing these substances will worsen the symptoms of patients with chronic cardiac or pulmonary diseases, but the relationship between air pollution and the actual production of lung disease in previously healthy individuals is less clear. Research on this question is underway and may define the connection in the future. At the moment it is thought that cigarette smoking damages the lungs and causes more disease than air pollution. Secondhand smoke, smoke passively inhaled by nonsmokers, may also turn out to be harmful for people in close contact with heavy smokers.

Not only industrial processes cause lung disease. Dusts containing plant or animal proteins —

Danger may lurk even in this rural scene, depicted by sixteenth-century Flemish painter Pieter Bruegel. Farmer's lung is a respiratory disease caused by a reaction to spores found in moldy hay.

In the early days of cotton manufacture, workers were liable to suffer from byssinosis, a lung disease caused by the inhalation of cotton dust. Continued exposure caused permanent damage to the lungs.

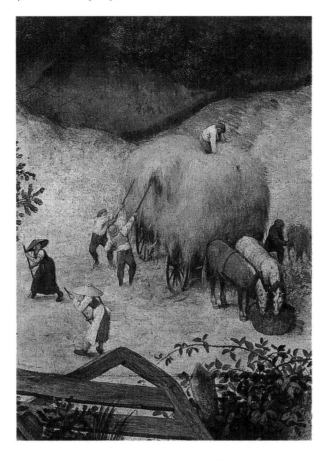

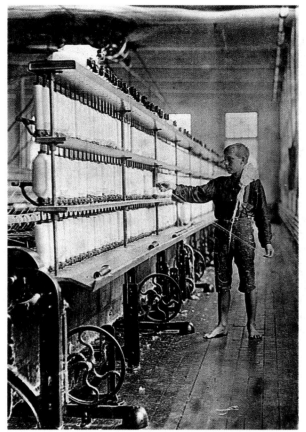

organic dusts — cause a type of illness known as hypersensitivity pneumonitis, or extrinsic allergic alveolitis. These names reflect the fact that an allergic reaction to the organic dust is set off usually four to six hours after its inhalation. Unlike the asthmatic reaction, with wheezing and airflow obstruction, this takes the form of a type of pneumonia. If a person has recurrent exposure to the offending dust, he may suffer a chronic scarring (or fibrotic) type of pneumonitis.

Farmer's lung, caused by the inhalation of dust from moldy hay containing a bacterium called *Thermophilic actinomycetes*, was the first of these diseases to be well understood. The organisms grow in the warm, wet centers of bales of stored hay. When the hay is "pitched" and disturbed, clouds of white dust containing billions of spores are released and inhaled by the farm worker who, some four to six hours later, may develop fever, a dry cough, shortness of breath and chills. If a

pulmonary function test were to be performed on the farm worker at this time, he or she would show a reduction in vital capacity.

Treatment of hypersensitivity pneumonitis is to remove the offending dust from the patient's environment or, if that is not possible, to remove the patient from the environment containing the dust. Corticosteroid medications can also be helpful. Similar diseases caused by organic dust are bird fancier's lung, which affects pigeon or parakeet handlers, and bagassosis, from the inhalation of dust from baggasse, the fibrous residue of sugarcane.

One that may affect office workers is hypersensitivity pneumonitis owing to the presence of bacteria in air conditioners and humidifiers. The total list of possible offending agents is long, and the key to diagnosing these disorders is a thorough investigation of the occupational, travel and environmental history of the patient.

There is a form of asthma, known as occupational asthma, which is precipitated by an allergen in the workplace. For example, bakers and millworkers may develop asthma due to allergy to grain dust; woodworkers can react to wood dust; and toluene diisocyanate, a substance found in plastics and some building materials, is also a potential allergen.

Pulmonary Vascular Disease

Alterations in the ratio between blood flow and ventilation in the lungs can affect overall gas exchange. Diseases of the pulmonary blood vessels are common and important causes of both acute and chronic lung complaints.

In pulmonary embolism, the most dramatic example of acute pulmonary vascular disease, a blood clot migrates, usually from leg veins, through the heart into the pulmonary arteries. Of the 600,000 cases of the disease every year in the United States, pulmonary embolism may be the sole cause of death in about 100,000 of these and a major contributing factor in another 100,000.

Blood clots that end up in the lungs usually form in the veins of the legs or pelvis. Predisposing factors, such as excessive clotting ability of the blood, injury or abnormality in the wall of a leg vein and stoppage of the blood are usually present before pulmonary embolism develops. A clot in the deep veins of the leg — deep venous thrombosis — may or may not be clinically apparent before a pulmonary embolism.

When a clot breaks loose from a leg vein and migrates through the heart to the lungs, an acute, dramatic set of symptoms develops. The patient develops severe chest pain, which worsens on breathing in, shortness of breath and rapid and sometimes irregular heart rate. The patient may also cough and spit blood. With severe massive pulmonary emboli, the blood flow out of the heart into the lungs is obstructed so dramatically that the patient may suffer a fall in blood pressure, loss of consciousness or cardiac arrest.

If small pulmonary emboli reach the peripheral areas of the lung, lung destruction may develop which usually causes bloody fluid to accumulate in the pleural space. Although small pulmonary emboli may not even be noticed, if they are recurrent, they may eventually obstruct so many small pulmonary vessels that the pulmonary pressure increases and puts a strain on the heart.

Pulmonary embolism is treated by administering medications to inhibit blood clotting or to dissolve blood clots. Sometimes, if anticlotting medicines do not work, or if they cannot be used because they have promoted bleeding, a filter is inserted into the large vein to the abdomen, the inferior vena cava, to prevent blood clots from migrating to the lungs.

Recognizing patients at risk and taking steps to decrease that risk can prevent pulmonary embolism. Nowadays, after surgery, patients are encouraged to get up and out of bed as soon as possible. Patients with heart failure or other illnesses requiring prolonged bed rest are often given small doses of anticlotting medicines to prevent pulmonary embolism.

Pulmonary Hypertension

The normal pulmonary circulation is a low pressure system. If pressure in the pulmonary arteries increases, the right side of the heart must work harder to pump blood through the lungs, and heart enlargement and failure result. This elevated pressure, or pulmonary hypertension, can stem from heart disease or from lung diseases that produce low blood oxygen levels, such as chronic bronchitis and emphysema (low oxygen levels make the pulmonary blood vessels narrow or constrict). Primary pulmonary hypertension is a rare disorder in which the lungs are normal, but the blood vessels in the lungs are scarred, narrowed and difficult to pump blood through. A progressive disease, it predominantly afflicts young women and may be fatal within a few years of diagnosis.

Fluid in the Lungs

Pulmonary edema means simply fluid in the lungs. Collection of fluid in the alveoli makes gas exchange extremely difficult and can be life threatening. Heart disease is the most common cause of pulmonary edema: when the heart muscle fails to pump blood effectively, fluid backs up into the lungs and floods the alveoli. This often happens after a massive heart attack, and the patient may cough up pink, frothy liquid.

Pulmonary edema can also develop in a person with normal heart and back pressure into the lungs;

For a variety of reasons, fluid can enter the lungs causing the condition termed pulmonary edema. The alveoli are flooded, as shown in this magnified section of lung tissue, and gas exchange is severely impaired.

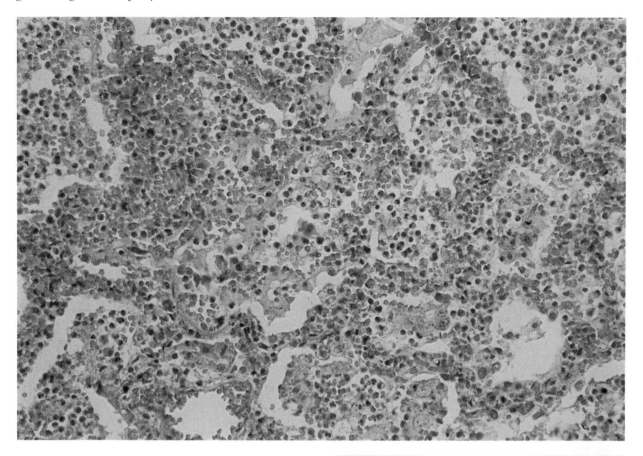

something happens that causes the pulmonary capillaries to leak fluid and protein material into the alveoli. This type of pulmonary edema results in what has been termed the adult respiratory distress syndrome (ARDS) and is a common cause of respiratory failure in patients with overwhelming, catastrophic illness. Such patients develop severe shortness of breath, and X rays of their chests show changes in the alveoli.

This fluid that leaks into the lungs in ARDS is not simply water, but is rich in proteins and often bloody. Flooding of the alveoli makes the lungs stiff and difficult to inflate, contributing to respiratory failure. The underlying illnesses linked with this condition include shock, massive trauma, overwhelming infection in the bloodstream, certain drug overdoses and, in some cases, head injuries. ARDS has also been named "shock lung," "traumatic wet lung" or "Da Nang lung" after the cases first noted during the Vietnam war. Another

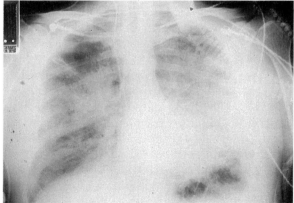

A form of pulmonary edema, adult respiratory distress syndrome is associated with extremely severe illness or trauma. Breathing becomes increasingly difficult and respiratory failure may ensue.

99

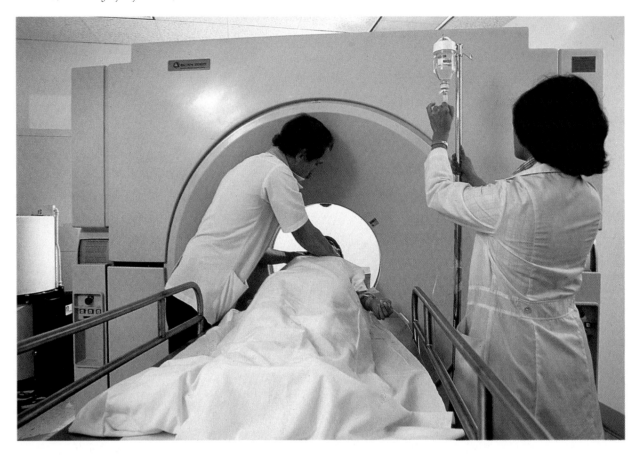

type of noncardiac pulmonary edema can be brought on by rapid ascent to high altitudes, and skiers and mountain climbers have been known to develop it.

Cardiogenic pulmonary edema can be treated by diuretics, medication to promote the excretion of excess fluid by the kidneys, and by drugs such as digitalis to improve the pumping ability of the heart. Morphine and other drugs that dilate the blood vessels can also be life saving in these cases.

Infections, shock, trauma, high altitude and the many other causes of noncardiac pulmonary edema may produce the condition through a variety of mechanisms, but all have in common leaking pulmonary capillaries. This type of edema is more difficult to manage than the cardiogenic and has a high mortality rate. Patients may be given life-support treatment by mechanical respirators, while their underlying illness, such as severe infection or hemorrhage, is treated. Diuretic medicines help prevent noncardiac pulmonary edema from worsening but do not reverse it in the way they do the cardiogenic type.

Symptoms of respiratory illness often play a prominent role in systemic diseases — those that affect the whole body. The exact cause of many of these systemic disorders is unknown, but infection, altered immunological responses and environmental factors have all been considered.

One such disease is sarcoidosis, which affects many organs of the body with changes similar to those caused by TB, although no infecting organism has been found to be responsible for these changes. Formation of fleshy lesions similar to those in TB, but without caseous, or cheesy, material in their centers, is characteristic of sarcoidosis. If the disease progresses, the lung may become scarred.

Most common in young adults in their twenties and thirties, sarcoidosis occurs in all countries,

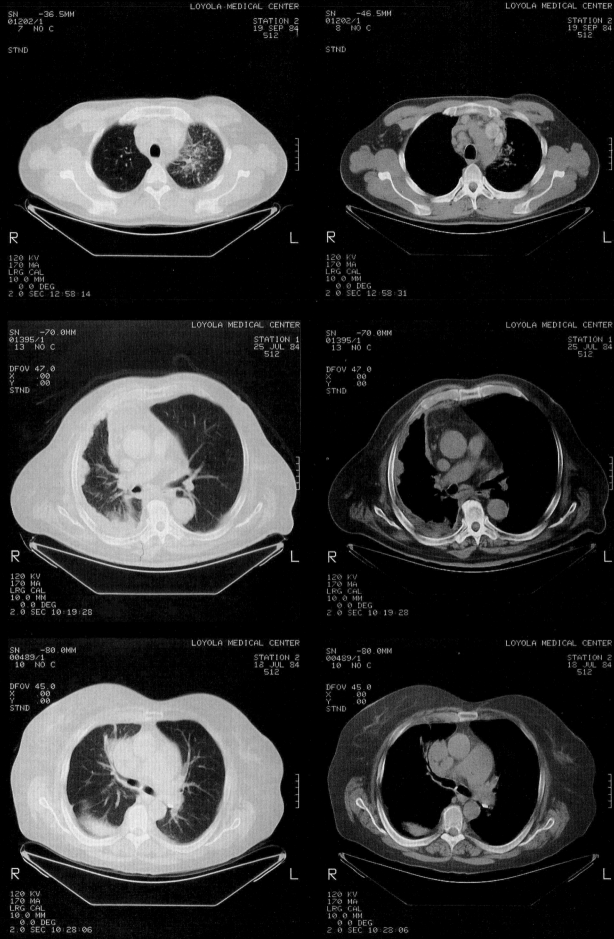

WHY START A LIFE UNDER A CLOUD?

Smoking is harmful to your baby's health. Quit for both of you. For help call your American Cancer Society.

AMERICAN CANCER SOCIETY

Expecting a baby means breathing for two. Cigarette smoking by the pregnant woman is particularly hazardous since it causes a significant decrease in the amount of oxygen available to the baby. The toxic compounds the smoke contains also have side effects which can damage the baby. Women who smoke during pregnancy have a higher than average risk of miscarriage and premature delivery, and their children may have twice as many respiratory problems and illnesses as children of nonsmokers.

ethnic groups and races. In the United States, it is most common among blacks, affecting black females three times more often than males. It may have few obvious symptoms and, in many cases, would go unnoticed if not for an abnormality picked up on a screening chest X ray. Although the lungs are involved in 90 percent of sarcoidosis patients, only about 25 percent show respiratory symptoms. Common symptoms include a mild cough, shortness of breath on exertion, low-grade fever, and weight loss.

Patients with sarcoidosis do not react normally to tests of the functioning of their natural immune system. Skin tests usually positive in normal people may produce no reaction in sarcoid patients. However, when a dose of material prepared from the spleen of a patient with sarcoidosis is injected under the skin, a typical granuloma will form in sarcoid patients, but not in normal patients. Known as the Kveim-Siltzbach test after its two developers, this can be helpful in the diagnosis of sarcoidosis. These abnormal reactions of the immune system of sarcoid patients suggest that the disease may have its underlying cause in the immunity mechanism.

About two-thirds of patients with sarcoidosis recover completely. The rest are left with some degree of respiratory impairment if not prevented with treatment. Corticosteroids are an effective treatment for the disease, particularly when it does not clear up on its own and when the eyes, heart or central nervous system are involved.

Other systemic illnesses that affect the lungs include the arthritis and connective tissue groups of diseases. Rheumatoid arthritis, for example, is a deforming disease of the joints, but can also involve the lungs, causing nodules, pleural disease or scarring and fibrosis.

The lungs may seem to be prone to a depressing array of disorders and disease. Some of the causes of these, such as cigarette smoking and undue occupational hazards, we can take steps to avoid. Others, such as air pollution and infection, we cannot always guard against. However, a consciousness of the normal healthy functioning of the respiratory system and regular health screening can help to diagnose any disorder in its early stages and greatly improve the chances of successful treatment.

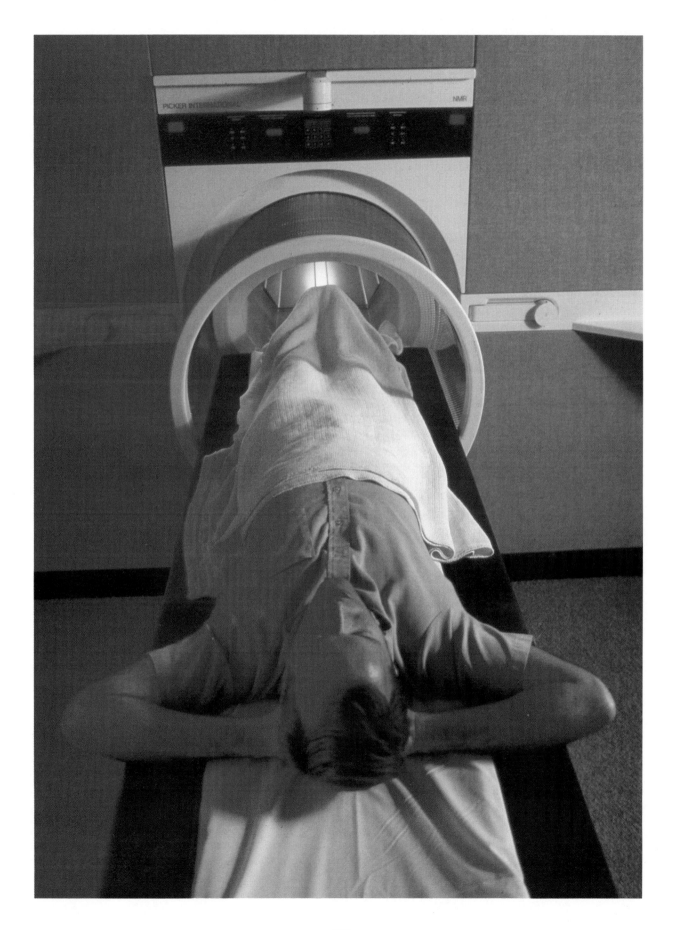

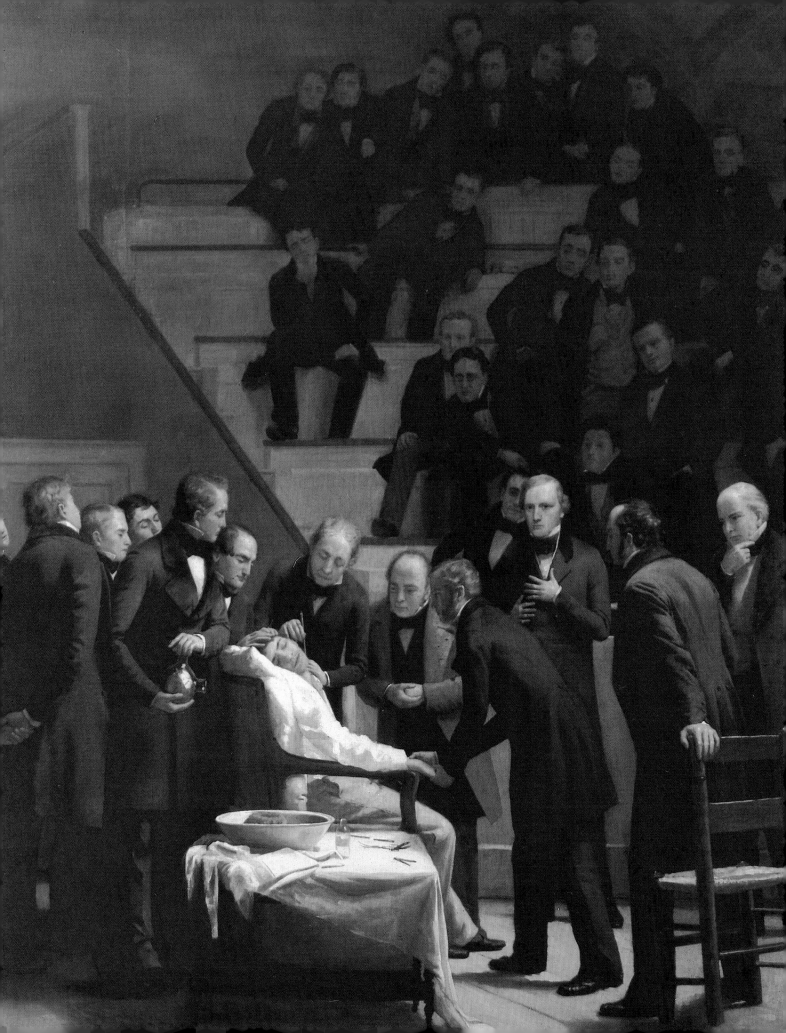

Chapter 6

Technology Takes Over

Without anesthesia, modern surgery would not be possible. A boil could be lanced or even a limb amputated, but only to save life and causing incalculable agonies in the process. Surgery for hernias, appendicitis, gall stones, duodenal ulcers, let alone cardiac surgery and neurosurgery, could not exist. The relevance of anesthesia to the subject of respiration is that, until recently, the only way in which anesthesia could be administered was via the lungs: an anesthetic vapor is inhaled and taken up into the bloodstream. Now, anesthesia can also be induced by injection.

Before the introduction of anesthesia in the nineteenth century, attempts were made to relieve the pain of surgical operations by administering alcohol — so that the patient was drunk to the point of stupor — or by using narcotics. For over two thousand years, opium has been known to act as a narcotic, but it was probably first used to blunt the pain of surgery in the ninth century A.D., as the main component of a soporific sponge. Steeped in the juices of the opium poppy and other medicinal herbs, such as mandragora, cicuta and hyoscyamus (known today as scopolamine), these sponges were held over the face of the patient who inhaled the vapor. Opium vapor was taken into the lungs and diffused across the alveolar membrane in the same way as oxygen, causing drowsiness.

Variations in the potency of these soporific sponges led to overdosage and many deaths, and their use was abandoned in the seventeenth century. Only in 1805, when the German pharmacist Friedrich Serturnier isolated the main alkaloid from the opium poppy, did opiate administration become possible on a scientific basis. The alkaloid was named morphine after Morpheus, the Roman god of sleep and dreams.

Although Joseph Priestley discovered nitrous oxide, the first of the anesthetic gases, in 1772, its analgesic properties were realized by Humphry Davy (1778–1829) only in 1799. Davy suggested that

The excitement and drama surrounding the first successful demonstration of ether anesthesia is evident in this painting (1882) by Robert Hinckley. The operation on the patient's jaw was performed by John Collins Warren in 1846 at the Massachusetts General Hospital. Known as the ether dome, the operating theater still stands in that hospital.

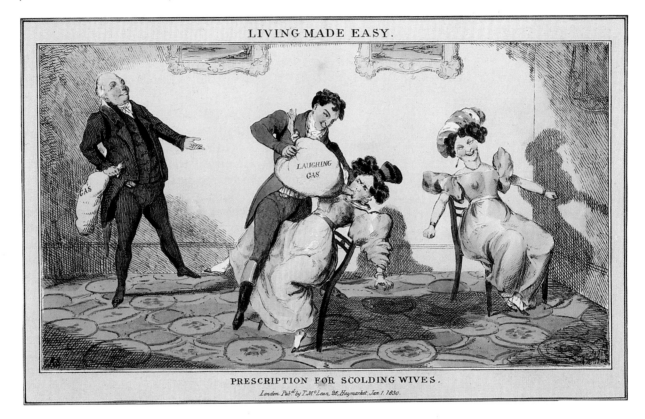

LIVING MADE EASY.

PRESCRIPTION FOR SCOLDING WIVES.

London. Pub.^d by T. McLean, 26, Haymarket, Jan. 1, 1830.

such gases might be used to relieve the pain of surgical operations, and it was he who gave nitrous oxide the name of laughing gas — because it literally caused patients to laugh and feel happy. Throughout the nineteenth century, nitrous oxide and sulfuric ether provided a somewhat dangerous source of amusement at parties. At these so-called ether frolics, partygoers breathed the gases to the point of pleasurable intoxication.

The First Anesthetics

In 1844, Horace Wells, a dentist from Connecticut, started using nitrous oxide to relieve the pain of tooth extraction. A year later he demonstrated his method at Harvard Medical School, but the patient complained of pain, and Wells was considered a fraud. Another dentist, William Morton (1819–68), and his former lecturer Charles Jackson, suggested the use of ether as an anesthetic for surgical operations to John Collins Warren (1778–1856), a famous Boston surgeon. As a result, the first surgical operation under ether anesthesia took

place in the Massachusetts General Hospital in 1846, when Warren removed a tumor from the jaw of a patient; both Morton and Jackson were present at the operation.

Two other dentists had used ether some four years previously but, since they did not publish their findings until much later, the credit for the introduction of anesthesia must go to Morton and Jackson. While the use of this new method spread rapidly on both sides of the Atlantic, despite the objections of the conservative elements in the medical world, its three proponents, Wells, Morton and Jackson contested the credit for its introduction. All died in unfortunate circumstances: Wells became a chloroform addict, was jailed for spraying a prostitute with sulfuric acid and subsequently committed suicide; Morton died a pauper and Jackson became insane.

Chloroform was introduced into anesthetic practice by James Simpson (1811–70), a British anesthetist who used it in midwifery, for which he was strongly attacked on religious grounds.

William Morton

Pioneer of Anesthesia

In the second quarter of the nineteenth century, ether frolics and nitrous oxide parties were all the rage, particularly in the United States, but these gases were not yet taken seriously by the medical profession. Some physicians, however, such as Crawford Long and dentist Horace Wells, noticed that the wild partygoers seemed insensible to any bruises or injuries they sustained while under the influence of the substances.

While Long and Wells recognized the potential of ether and nitrous oxide as agents of pain relief, it was another dentist, William Morton, who successfully demonstrated to the scientific world the use of ether as an anesthetic for surgical operations.

Born in 1819, in Charlton, Massachusetts, Morton is believed to have trained at the Baltimore College of Dentistry — the first dental school in America — although little is known of his early life. He had a brief partnership with Horace Wells, whose enthusiastic search for a painless method of tooth extraction was undoubtedly of great influence.

In 1845, soon after establishing his own practice in Boston, Morton helped to arrange an operation at the Massachusetts General Hospital during which Wells might demonstrate the

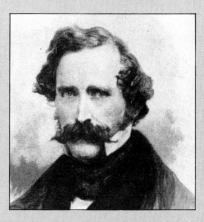

anesthetic properties of nitrous oxide. The demonstration was a failure, but, despite the general skepticism, Morton was still convinced that effective anesthesia was possible.

With the help of his former teacher, Boston chemist Charles Jackson, Morton learned that ether had greater possibilities than nitrous oxide. He began to experiment on animals, on himself and his assistants, using a handkerchief saturated with ether. Inhaling the fumes in this way did not always achieve the desired loss of sensibility and, with the help of an instrument maker, Morton developed a form of inhaler.

Having successfully extracted a tooth from a patient anesthetized with ether, William Morton was ready to introduce his method of anesthesia to the world.

In 1846, Morton arranged with surgeon John Collins Warren to administer ether to a young man in need of surgery. The demonstration, like that by Wells, took place at the Massachusetts General Hospital, but this time it was a success. Warren himself turned to the assembled company and said: "Gentlemen, this is no humbug."

Ether anesthesia then quickly gained acceptance in the medical world. So fast did the news spread that only a few months after the Boston operation British surgeon Robert Lister employed the ether technique in a painless and successful amputation operation in London.

Yet Morton gained little reward for his work. His attempts to patent the technique and claim for himself the credit for the discovery of anesthesia resulted in costly legal actions by Jackson and Wells. He neglected his work, failed to develop his discovery and spent the rest of his life fighting to secure some financial reward. He died penniless in New York on July 15, 1868, the victim of a stroke, brought on, it is said, by reading an article supporting the claims of Charles Jackson.

Elected posthumously in 1920 to the Hall of Fame for Great Americans, Morton is remembered as a pioneer of anesthesia who brought to the attention of the world the means of painless surgery.

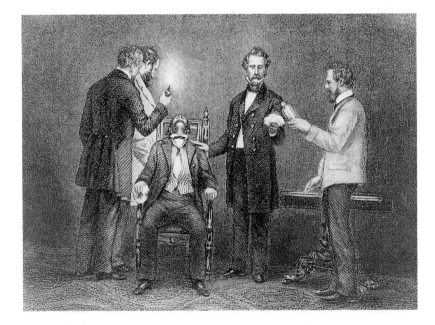

Theologians quoted the Old Testament as proof that childbirth was meant to cause pain.

> Unto the woman He said, I will greatly multiply thy sorrow and thy conception; in sorrow thou shalt bring forth children
>
> (Genesis 3, 16)

John Snow (1813–58) was the first great scientist to work in the field of anesthesia; in 1847 he published the first scientific textbook on the subject, *On the Inhalation of Ether in Surgical Operations*. Later he abandoned the use of ether for the newer chloroform and, having invented a known percentage chloroform inhaler, made the first scientific administrations of an anesthetic. When Snow administered the drug to Queen Victoria during the birth of her eighth child, in 1853, chloroform achieved respectability. Queen Victoria said: "Doctor Snow administered that blessed chloroform and the effect was soothing, quieting and delightful beyond measure."

Chloroform soon became widely used as an anesthetic. However, uncontrolled administration too often led to overdosage and death, due to decreased cardiac and respiratory function. There was certainly a need for a more controlled and scientific method of administering these potent and dangerous vapors.

Joseph T. Clover (1825–82) invented a new inhaler for chloroform administration. This was basically a large bag containing 4.5 percent of chloroform in air; the patient inhaled the chloroform through tubing attached to the bag. In another method of administering chloroform or ether, developed about the same time, a wire mask covered with gauze wadding was used; the liquid to be vaporized was dropped onto the wadding and the mask held over the patient's face.

The Stages of Anesthesia

The same anesthetic agents remained in use for decades. In 1920, the American anesthetist Arthur E. Guedel (1883–1956) published his first paper on the signs of anesthesia, research findings that he subsequently developed into the classic stages of anesthesia. His description concerns ether anesthesia but applies to other inhaled anesthetics.

The first stage is analgesia; responses to pain are reduced but the patient is still cooperative. The second stage, beginning when the patient loses consciousness, is that of excitement and uninhibited responses and may include struggling and vomiting. Surgical anesthesia, stage three, starts when this excitement stage ceases and regular, automatic respiration commences. During this stage, surgery can take place. As anesthesia

John Snow

Anesthetist to Royalty

A few drops of chloroform on the corner of a royal handkerchief were sufficient to change the course of anesthesia once and for all. When John Snow administered the anesthetic to Queen Victoria at the birth of Prince Leopold in 1853, he ensured public acceptance of anesthesia as a means of pain relief in childbirth.

The eldest son of a farmer, John Snow was born in 1813 in York, England. Little is known of his early life, but at the age of fourteen he became apprentice to a surgeon in Newcastle-upon-Tyne, England. Snow worked hard, and when the first cholera epidemic struck England he gained a deep interest in and lasting knowledge of this disease which he would later help to conquer.

Moving to London in 1836, he studied medicine and later established himself as a general practitioner. Snow was a tireless, conscientious doctor, but his devotion to his patients did not keep him from scientific investigation. He studied asphyxia, resuscitation and other aspects of the physiology of respiration and has the reputation of being one of the few men in the first half of the nineteenth century to do original medical research.

Having heard of the historic experiments made in the United

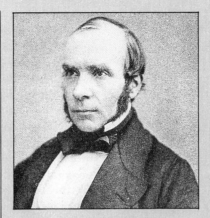

States with ether, Snow soon invented a means of improving the reliability of ether administration. He demonstrated his method to dental surgeons who were so impressed that Snow was much in demand to administer ether during operations.

When another British anesthetist, James Simpson, introduced chloroform anesthesia in 1847, Snow was quick to appreciate its advantages and drawbacks. Using his experience with ether, he developed equipment for delivering low and exact percentages of chloroform. Unlike ether, chloroform is a dangerous and volatile chemical, which, in the wrong hands, can easily be fatal. Snow, however, after detailed research was able to tame it to some extent, and lay down strict guidelines for the safer administration of chloroform anasthesia.

Soon after its introduction, a great controversy broke out over the use of chloroform. With other advocates, Snow battled against considerable religious and medical opposition, particularly in the field of midwifery. In 1853, Snow's opponents learned to their dismay that he had administered chloroform to Queen Victoria during the birth of Prince Leopold, and that she was extremely pleased with the effects. A royal precedent had been set and, almost overnight, the use of chloroform to reduce the pains of childbirth became every mother's right and every doctor's duty.

John Snow's achievements were not only in the field of anesthesia. He made a fundamental contribution to the understanding of the transmission of infectious diseases when he proved that cholera was transmitted by water infected by fecal matter. This was confirmed in 1884 when Robert Koch identified the organism that caused cholera.

Victim of a cerebral hemorrhage, John Snow died at the age of forty-five. That year, the British medical journal, the *Lancet*, which only a few years previously had refused to believe Snow had given chloroform to Queen Victoria, described him as the outstanding physician of his day.

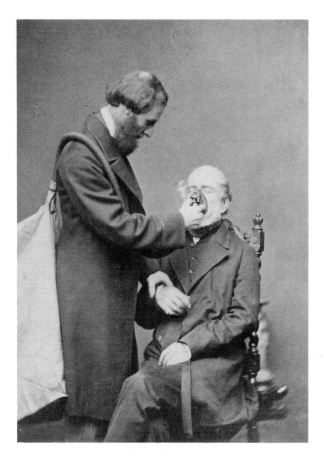

*Early use of anesthesia caused many
deaths from overdosage.
Nineteenth-century anesthetist
Joseph T. Clover attempted to
improve the controlled application of
anesthetic agents with his invention
of an inhaler. A mix of chloroform
and air was prepared in advance, so
that the exact proportions were
known, and was contained in a large
bag carried on the anesthetist's
shoulder. The patient inhaled the
vapors through tubing from the bag.*

deepens, the functioning of the muscles of respiration is increasingly impaired until paralysis stops respiration. At this point of overdosage, stage four, the diaphragm stops moving, respiration and all other reflex activity stops and is followed by paralysis and death unless there is medical intervention.

Induction of anesthesia with ether or chloroform is not a pleasant experience for the patient. Both gases have an extremely pungent vapor, which the patient may have to inhale for several minutes while the anesthetic passes across the alveolar membrane into the bloodstream and then to the brain. Anesthesia has been made much less unpleasant, however, by the introduction of intravenous anesthetic agents. Following a single injection of such a substance into the patient's vein, anesthesia can be induced within ten seconds, thus compressing the early stages into a much shorter time than previously possible.

Short-acting barbiturates are the drugs most commonly used for the intravenous induction of anesthesia, the first two to be introduced, in the 1920s, being sodium amytal and pentobarbitone (Nembutal). Sodium pentothal (thiopental, thiopentone) was synthesized in 1932 and first administered in 1934 by Ralph Waters, the father of modern American anesthetic practice.

Intravenous Anesthesia

Induction of anesthesia with thiopental is pleasant, and after the injection many patients are asleep before they can count to ten. In a typical anesthetic today, an intravenous injection of thiopental rapidly takes the patient to stage three, after which he breathes a combination of nitrous oxide, oxygen and one of the newer volatile agents (halothane, enflurane or isoflurane) which have supplanted ether and chloroform.

After induction, anesthesia must be continued with an inhalational agent because a single dose of thiopental is effective for only about five minutes. Its duration of action is limited not by its excretion from the body, but by its redistribution, as the blood circulates, to muscle and fat and away from the brain where it exerts its action. If the induction dose is repeated several times, the body stores become full of thiopental which cannot be redistributed away from the brain, thus prolonging its effectiveness. Some residual effect of thiopental explains why many people feel sleepy for a prolonged period after anesthesia. Both thiopental and the volatile agents can cause nausea.

Anesthetic agents act on the nerve cells of both the peripheral and central nervous systems, but the question of exactly how they produce their effect is one that has long perplexed scientists. The effects of anesthetics are apparently concentrated on specialized areas of the nerve cells. One early observation was that anesthetics were particularly soluble in fat, so would be readily absorbed by cells, including those of the central nervous system. Once absorbed, the anesthetic molecules disturb the transmission of nervous impulses. Another theory is that anesthesia is the result of interaction between the anesthetic molecules and the water found within the cell. None of the present theories about anesthetic action fully explains all the experimental observations, however, and, despite the fact that they are in daily use, understanding of the way in which anesthetic agents work is incomplete.

Muscle Relaxants

Using the anesthetic techniques described, it can be difficult for the surgeon to gain access to certain parts of the body; for example, access to the upper abdomen and thorax is limited unless the muscles of respiration are almost paralyzed. The depth of anesthesia required to achieve the necessary degree of muscular relaxation is close to overdosage, so, in such instances, another group of drugs is used to induce muscle relaxation. A plant used for centuries by South American Indian tribes to poison arrows here comes to the aid of modern anesthesia.

Sir Walter Raleigh (1552–1618), Elizabethan adventurer and explorer, was the first westerner to describe this arrow poison, known as curare, which was prepared from an infusion of the bark of a plant named *Strychnos toxifera*. Some three hundred years after Raleigh, an English explorer, Charles Waterton (1783–1865), went to South America to gather specimens of the plant. Having prepared an infusion, Waterton injected a donkey with some poison and, when it appeared to have died, made

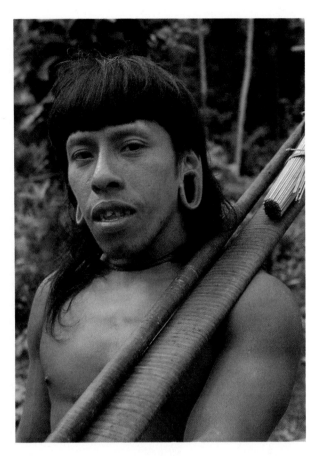

For centuries, the Indians of the tropical forests of South America have used curare, a substance prepared from the bark of a plant, to poison arrows; the effect of curare is to paralyze the muscles of the victim. In the nineteenth century, an English explorer collected specimens of the plant to investigate its potential in medicine. If curare is administered to an anesthetized patient, all muscular activity ceases, and surgical access, to the chest for example, is dramatically improved, without the need to administer dangerously large doses of anesthetic. However, once the respiratory muscles are paralyzed by curare, ventilation must be continued artificially by machine.

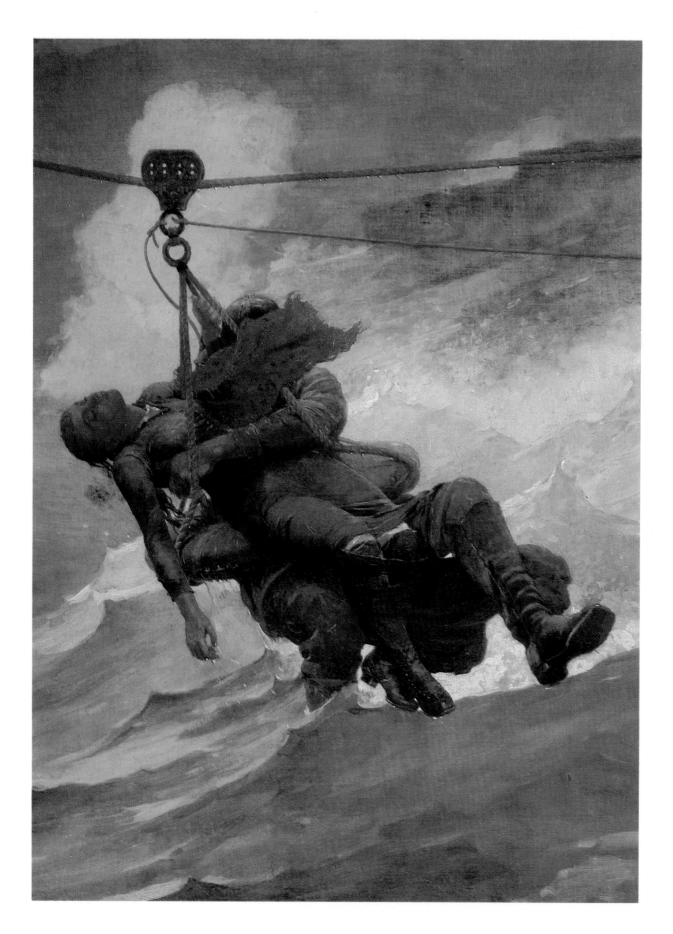

The Life Line *by Winslow Homer depicts a dramatic sea rescue. Any person who has been close to drowning will need resuscitation, and immediate attention must be given to restoring breathing.*

Most drownings occur as a result of inhaling large amounts of water. The airways and alveoli flood, preventing respiration. The effect on the lungs is illustrated in this nineteenth-century drawing.

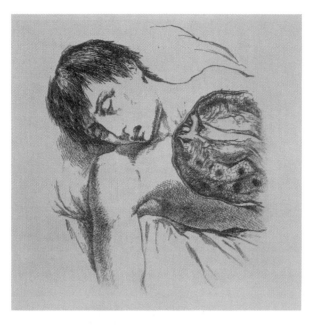

an incision in its trachea and inflated the lungs with a pair of bellows for four hours. The donkey made a complete recovery, proving that the action of the curare was to paralyze, not kill.

Curare acts by blocking the nerve-muscle junctions. There is a substance in nerve cells, acetyl choline, which conveys signals from nerves to muscles, telling them to contract. By occupying the acetyl choline receptors on the muscles, curare stops any messages from the nerves getting through. All the muscles are then paralyzed. When curare is given to a patient under anesthesia, surgical access is improved because the respiratory muscles cease to function — but the patient stops breathing. Two other advances were necessary before curare and similar drugs, known as the neuromuscular blocking agents, could become part of the anesthetist's armory.

Devices had to be developed to allow automatic ventilation of the lungs — and there had to be easy access to the lungs to allow ventilation to be carried out. The tracheotomy and bellows method used by Waterton on his donkey was certainly not appropriate for every surgical procedure requiring muscle relaxation.

Waterton was not, incidentally, the first to undertake artificial respiration. In the Old Testament, in the Second book of Kings, the prophet Elisha resuscitated an apparently dead Shunammite: "And he went up, and lay upon the child, and put his mouth upon his mouth and his eyes upon his eyes, and his hands upon his hands: and he stretched himself upon the child; and the flesh of the child waxed warm ... and the child sneezed seven times, and the child opened his eyes."

Techniques of Artificial Respiration

The first serious attempts to consider the problem of artificial respiration were made in 1769, when the Society for the Recovery of Drowned Persons was formed in Amsterdam with the purpose of discovering effective means of resuscitation. An English surgeon, John Hunter, proposed the use of bellows and invented a pair of two-way bellows for the purpose. In 1837 this method was superseded, when the Royal Humane Society in London recommended artificial respiration by external compression of the chest wall, a technique

that remained in use until the late 1950s, when it was shown that actually blowing into the lungs was more effective.

The suggestion that intermittent positive pressure ventilation — blowing gases into the lungs — might be applicable in anesthesia was first made by American anesthetist Ralph Waters in 1932. He realized that squeezing the reservoir bag (part of the tubing on the anesthetic machinery) might be a useful way of preventing lung collapse during thoracic surgery. Only a little of this auxiliary reserve of gas is normally taken, but if the gas in the bag is deliberately squeezed into the patient's lungs, they are forced to inflate. This method was first used to treat patients with respiratory failure during the Scandinavian polio epidemic of 1952. Medical students worked in eight-hour shifts for periods of up to three months to keep patients alive by repeatedly squeezing the reservoir bag.

More recently, mechanical devices for artificial ventilation have been developed to replace relays of medical students. Methods of maintaining artificial respiration fall into four categories: first, manual compression of the chest wall; second, gas pressure applied to the upper respiratory tract; third, pressure changes applied to the trunk but not to the head; fourth, displacement of the abdominal contents lying under the diaphragm.

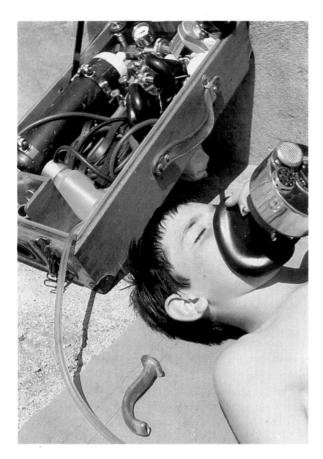

Ultimately there are only two causes of death—cardiac arrest and the cessation of breathing. In any accident, the first priority must be to check the victim's breathing, before any attention is given to bleeding wounds or broken bones. Deprived of oxygen for as little as four minutes, the brain may suffer permanent damage. Consequently all personnel who deal with emergencies carry oxygen equipment and are trained in resuscitation techniques.

The first category, manual compression of the chest wall, includes techniques of artificial respiration such as the Silvester method: the lower portion of the chest is compressed and the arms moved backward and outward to cause the lungs to draw air in. Such emergency methods have been superseded by mouth-to-mouth resuscitation — one way of applying gas pressure to the upper respiratory tract. All modern forms of ventilation during anesthesia and intensive care also work on the principle of applying gas pressure to the upper airways, but by means of machines.

These life-support machines provide intermittent positive pressure ventilation (IPPV) and are an essential part of the equipment of intensive care units. IPPV is carried out by connecting the patient's upper airway to a machine containing bellows filled with respirable gas. During inspiration, the bellows contract — either mechanically or driven by gas pressure from outside — and air is forced into the patient's lungs. Breathing out is accomplished passively, simply by allowing the elastic recoil of the lungs to expel the air.

The great advantage of IPPV is that the patient is free of all apparatus and is connected to the machine only by the tube running from his upper airway. The machinery controlling ventilation is thus separate from the patient, allowing free access to the surgeon during anesthesia, or to nursing staff if it is in use as a life support in an intensive care unit. But the way in which the patient is attached to the machine is also the major disadvantage of IPPV. Since ventilation depends on positive pressure being applied to the patient's airway, sealed access to the airway is required. Either a tube with a cuff around it is placed in the trachea via the mouth or nose and the cuff expanded to seal access — the method used during anesthesia — or a cuffed tube is placed in the trachea through the neck by surgery, a tracheotomy. Both solutions have their complications; cuffed endotracheal tubes can be used for only a limited period, and a patient with a tracheotomy is unable to speak.

The Iron Lung

Tank ventilators, or iron lungs, apply pressure to the outside of the chest wall; Professor P. Drinker of Harvard designed the first power-driven tank ventilator in 1928. The patient is placed in a rigid metal tank from which only his head protrudes, and the tank is connected to mechanically operated bellows. The tank is rendered airtight around the patient's neck by a flexible padded collar, split into two sections. During inspiration the bellows expand and suck air out of the tank. The pressure surrounding the lungs becomes less than that of the air outside in the atmosphere, the lungs expand, and air is drawn in from the outside. During expiration, the bellows contract, the pressure in the tank returns to that of the atmosphere, and the elastic recoil of the lungs makes them contract so that air flows out passively.

Although tank ventilators are cumbersome and difficult to use, they still retain a place in modern medicine and are used in long-term care of patients with severe weakness of the respiratory muscles. Such patients, with respiratory weakness following polio for example, may be able to breathe adequately when awake but require the assistance of a tank ventilator when asleep. A modification of the tank ventilator is the cuirass — basically a rigid shell over the thorax and abdomen with an airtight seal at either end. Less efficient than the tank, the cuirass can be used only to assist the respiration of partially paralyzed patients.

Mechanical displacement of structures under the diaphragm is accomplished using a motor-driven rocking bed. In the head-up position, the abdominal contents are displaced downward; the resulting downward movement of the diaphragm sucks some air into the lungs. When the patient is tipped head-down, expiration occurs by the reverse process.

Developments in endotracheal intubation — the placing of a tube in the trachea — accompanied advances in mechanical ventilation. A cuffed tube in the trachea provided the sealed access required for IPPV and also allowed shared access to the airway when oral or facial surgery was being carried out. Endotracheal intubation was pioneered by two British anesthesiologists Sir Ivor Magill and Edgar Stanley Rowbotham, at the end of World War I. Both worked with one of the pioneers of plastic surgery, Harold Gillies, in the Hospital for Facial and Jaw Injuries, treating soldiers injured in battle.

Because of the nature of the surgery, it was obviously impossible to hold a mask in place to

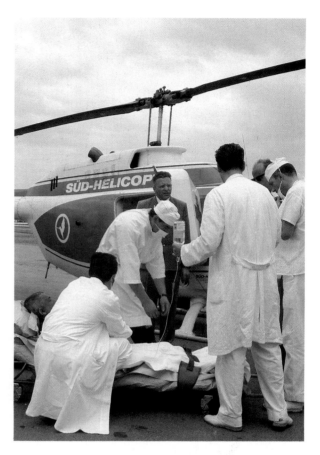

Modern technology makes a dramatic difference to a patient in severe respiratory distress, whether from illness or accident. Helicopters, equipped with full life-support machinery, can rush to the scene, and the patient's cardiac and respiratory systems can be maintained during the journey to hospital.

In order to gain surgical access to the heart, its action must cease and its functions be taken over by machinery. In a cardiopulmonary bypass operation, no blood flows through the heart or lungs but drains into tubes inserted into the veins carrying blood to the heart. A machine takes over the job of the lungs, and the blood circulation in the rest of the body continues as normal during the operation.

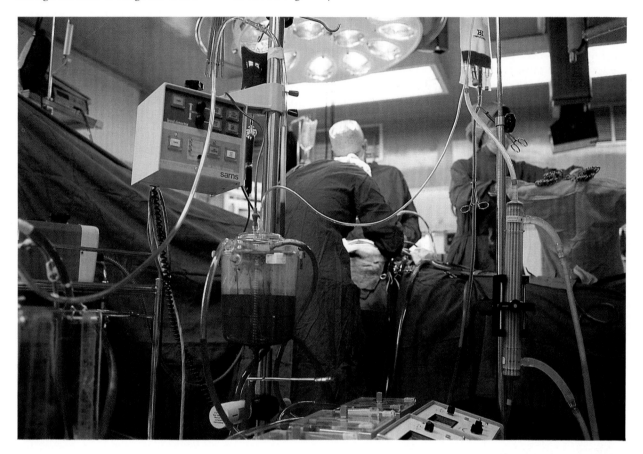

administer anesthetic. Instead, a narrow, hollow, gum-elastic tube was passed into the trachea, using a laryngoscope. A curved instrument with a light at one end, the laryngoscope, when inserted into the mouth, allowed vision of the larynx and also the passage of a tube into the trachea. Using a wider bore tube with an inflatable cuff around it, sealed access to the airway for attachment to an IPPV can be obtained.

Until recently, most endotracheal tubes were made of mineralized rubber, which, after a few hours, irritates the respiratory tract. Advances in plastics technology mean that today tubes are made of material such as polyvinyl chloride (PVC) and are less of an irritant.

With modern techniques of temporary paralysis of the subject and artificial ventilation with IPPV, concepts of anesthesia have moved away from Guedel's "stages" and toward a balanced approach. It is no longer necessary to take a patient to stage three anesthesia to enable abdominal surgery to take place. A number of drugs, each with its specific desired effect, can be used in smaller quantities, and the combination of them all gives a balanced anesthetic.

After induction of anesthesia with a short-acting barbiturate, such as thiopental, the anesthesiologist may choose a combination of a muscle relaxant, accompanied by nitrous oxide in oxygen, a small amount of an inhalational agent and perhaps an opioid analgesic. Such a mixture would guarantee lack of awareness and the suppression of reflexes during anesthesia. If the surgical procedure does not require muscle relaxation, the anesthesiologist may, after induction of anesthesia, allow the patient to breathe nitrous oxide in oxygen, with an inhalational agent to maintain anesthesia.

Whatever the technique employed, premedication can make the experience of anesthesia and surgery less unpleasant. Used only infrequently

116

during the first fifty years of anesthesia, "preliminary medication" was administered by 60 percent of all hospitals in the United States by 1914. The term "premedication" was first used in the American Journal of Surgery in 1920.

The history of premedication starts in 1869 with Claude Bernard, a French physiologist at the Sorbonne in Paris, who subdued animals with morphine prior to surgery. Some of his pupils then began to use morphine in an effort to reduce the amount of chloroform needed for deep anesthesia, but the practice continued only sporadically until the early twentieth century. The purpose of premedication is to administer drugs which facilitate the induction, maintenance and recovery from anesthesia. The ideal premedication reduces fear and anxiety before anesthesia and surgery and causes amnesia for the period of the induction of anesthesia. It can also reduce the secretion of saliva, which, in excess, can be troublesome during anesthesia. However, the use of such drying agents in premedication is currently questioned.

Typically, a premedication might be an intramuscular injection of an opioid, such as morphine or demerol, along with a drying agent, such as atropine or scopolamine, which also has some sedative properties. (Both scopolamine and thiopental have been used outside medicine as "truth serums" during interrogation.) Another approach to premedication is to give a tranquilizer, which allays anxiety and provides some amnesia. The drugs most commonly used for this purpose are the benzodiazepines, the best-known example of which is diazepam (Valium).

The development of the heart-lung machine is a recent technological advance that has affected anesthesia and surgery and is related to lung physiology. The idea of artificial organ perfusion — the artificial maintenance of an organ's blood circulation — does not, however, belong to the twentieth century. In 1812, physiologist J. J. C. Legallois wrote, "If one could substitute for the heart a kind of injection of artificial blood, either naturally or artificially made, one would succeed in maintaining alive indefinitely any part of the body whatsoever." The first experiments on organ perfusion were carried out by physiologist Charles Edward Brown-Séquard, who, in 1858, perfused the decapitated head of a dog with blood.

Experiments in producing oxygenated blood without its passing through the lungs progressed slowly and, because the investigators failed to realize the enormous surface area of blood that must be exposed if effective oxygenation is to occur, were unsuccessful. In 1865, physiologist Carl Ludwig tried shaking blood in a balloon filled with air; and, in 1890, other workers experimented with bubbling air through blood. In both instances the blood was adequately oxygenated but foamy. In 1885, Frey and Gruber tried exposing a thin film of blood to oxygen by allowing it to flow along the inside walls of a cylinder where it collected oxygen. The same principle was used by John Haysham Gibbon, who, in 1937, developed one of the first heart-lung machines, or oxygenators.

Bypassing Heart and Lungs

The main reason why early experiments on extracorporeal (outside the body) circulations failed was inability to stop blood coagulating in the circuit. The development of heparin, an agent which prevented blood clotting, and protamine, which reversed the action of heparin, combined with the advances in modern electronics and plastics, removed this difficulty. The first cardiopulmonary bypass operation on a human being, in which machinery took over the functions of both heart and lungs, was performed in 1951.

In the circuit used for cardiopulmonary bypass, plastic pipes are inserted into the superior and inferior vena cavae (the largest veins carrying blood to the heart) to drain the venous blood returning to the heart. Under the influence of gravity, the blood drains freely into the oxygenator which undertakes the function of the lungs, supplying oxygen to the blood and removing carbon dioxide. After oxygenation, the blood is pumped by a roller pump through a large pipe and back into the aorta. The heart is thereby isolated from the rest of the circulation, and no blood flows through the heart or lungs. The surgeon can then stop the heart beating and replace a valve, graft coronary arteries, implant an artificial pacemaker or carry out any other surgery.

The oxygenators used to provide gas exchange for cardiopulmonary bypass are of two types: those with a gas interface (screen or bubble) and those

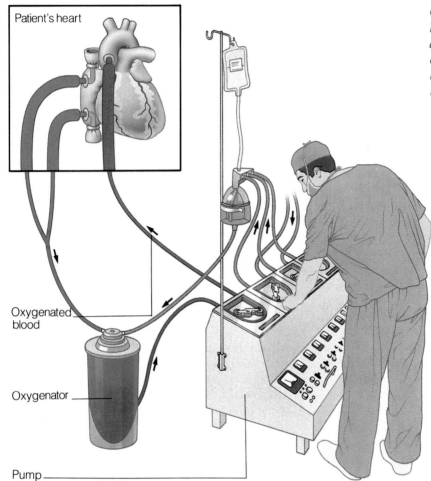

Patient's heart

Oxygenated blood

Oxygenator

Pump

Once the patient is connected to the heart-lung machine, blood is diverted into an oxygenator where oxygen is supplied and carbon dioxide removed. It is then pumped back into the body.

without (membrane). In a bubble oxygenator, the ventilating gases are passed through a perforated plate which produces bubbles about two to seven millimeters in diameter. As the bubbles pass through the blood in the reservoir, gas exchange takes place between the bubbles and the blood. Since it would be dangerous to introduce any air bubbles back into the arterial circulation because they block the arteries, and hence blood flow, the oxygenated blood must be meticulously debubbled and defoamed before being pumped back. Even so, this type of oxygenator can damage the blood over a period of time because of the mechanical trauma the bubbles cause to the red blood cells.

To overcome this difficulty, membrane oxygenators have been developed. In this type of machine, the blood passes between layers of semipermeable membrane, on the other side of which is gas, rich in oxygen, low in carbon dioxide. Gas, but not liquid, can move across the membrane and so gas exchange is achieved. The sheet of membrane is analogous to the thin walls of the alveoli in the lungs, and gases diffuse across in the same way.

Intensive Care and Respiratory Failure

With the development of highly technological methods of treatment, such as artificial ventilation of the lungs, and recent extraordinary advances in cardiac and neurosurgery, the need for specialized areas of patient care became clear. This need was first recognized during the Scandinavian polio epidemic of the 1950s, when units were set aside for the treatment of patients suffering the respiratory complications of the disease. Other specialized units were then set up, such as coronary care units.

From these specialized units came the concept of the Intensive Care Unit, or ICU, which provides more space, equipment and nursing care than may be available in other parts of a hospital. An ICU also provides a service which permits continuous observations of vital body functions, and it is equipped to support these functions artificially, should they fail. If a hospital has a particular commitment to treating cardiac patients, for example, or patients with respiratory failure, an ICU may become superspecialized, but generally the ICU cares for those who have any life-threatening disease process.

Respiratory failure is one reason for a patient requiring treatment in an ICU. There are two categories of respiratory failure: first, hypoxemic failure, when the blood is low in oxygen but there is no accompanying retention of carbon dioxide, and second, ventilatory failure, when not only do oxygen levels fall but carbon dioxide levels rise.

Hypoxemic failure occurs in the group of diseases affecting the lung alveoli or the spaces around them, known as the interstitium. It can follow pneumonia or occur as a result of left heart failure, when fluid leaks into the alveoli and interstitial spaces and interferes with gas transport. This can produce paroxysmal nocturnal dyspnea, a distressing condition in which the patient wakes at night unable to breathe because of the fluid that has collected in the lungs during sleep. If the affected person stands up, the fluid drains to the bottom of the lungs and breathing usually becomes easier. In hypoxemic lung failure, the problem is caused not by alteration in airway resistance but by a defect in ventilation–perfusion relationships, with an increase in physiological shuntings. This hypoxemia can be corrected by increasing the tension of the inspired oxygen.

By way of contrast, in ventilatory failure, the carbon dioxide level in the blood is increased in relation to a reduction in total ventilation. Problems in areas from the brain down to the lungs can be the cause of ventilatory failure. A tumor pressing on the brain stem — which contains the respiratory center — can affect respiration adversely, but it is more common for this type of respiratory failure to be produced by more general disturbances of brain function, leading to alterations in the state of consciousness and to coma. Drugs, particularly barbiturates and opioids such as morphine and heroin, may also decrease respiration by acting directly on the respiratory center. Damage to the spinal cord in the neck, as might occur after a road accident, can also affect the nerves to the muscles of respiration and lead to ventilatory failure; so can diseases such as polio.

Injury to the chest wall, affecting the firmness and mechanical uniformity of the thoracic cage, is another cause of ventilatory failure — again, chest injury is common in automobile accident victims. Diseases affecting the respiratory system itself, asthma, chronic bronchitis and emphysema for example, are perhaps the most common causes of ventilatory failure.

To treat respiratory failure, both the specific condition behind it and the failure of gas exchange must be corrected. Drugs may be used to control infections or, in asthma cases, to help widen the airways and make breathing easier. If the patient does not have enough oxygen in his blood, more must be supplied. In mild cases of hypoxemic failure, additional oxygen is given via plastic tubes inserted into the nostrils, or by a face mask over the nose and mouth. If this is insufficient, an endotracheal tube can be inserted and ventilation continued, using IPPV to help a patient through an acute episode of respiratory failure.

Being in an intensive care unit can be a very frightening experience. Imagine the feelings of a patient, who wakes after surgery and finds he is unable to speak because there is an endotracheal tube in his mouth, and that a machine is doing his breathing. Once recovered, however, thanks to the assistance of such a machine, the patient may reflect on the extraordinary advances in respiratory physiology of the last two hundred years. In the late eighteenth century Antoine Lavoisier and Joseph Priestley were unveiling the mysteries of lung function; now, there are sophisticated machines to perform that function for us. Intensive care units, and the apparatus they contain, are one of the major reasons patients are able to survive today's high technology medicine, and their importance is likely to expand in the years to come.

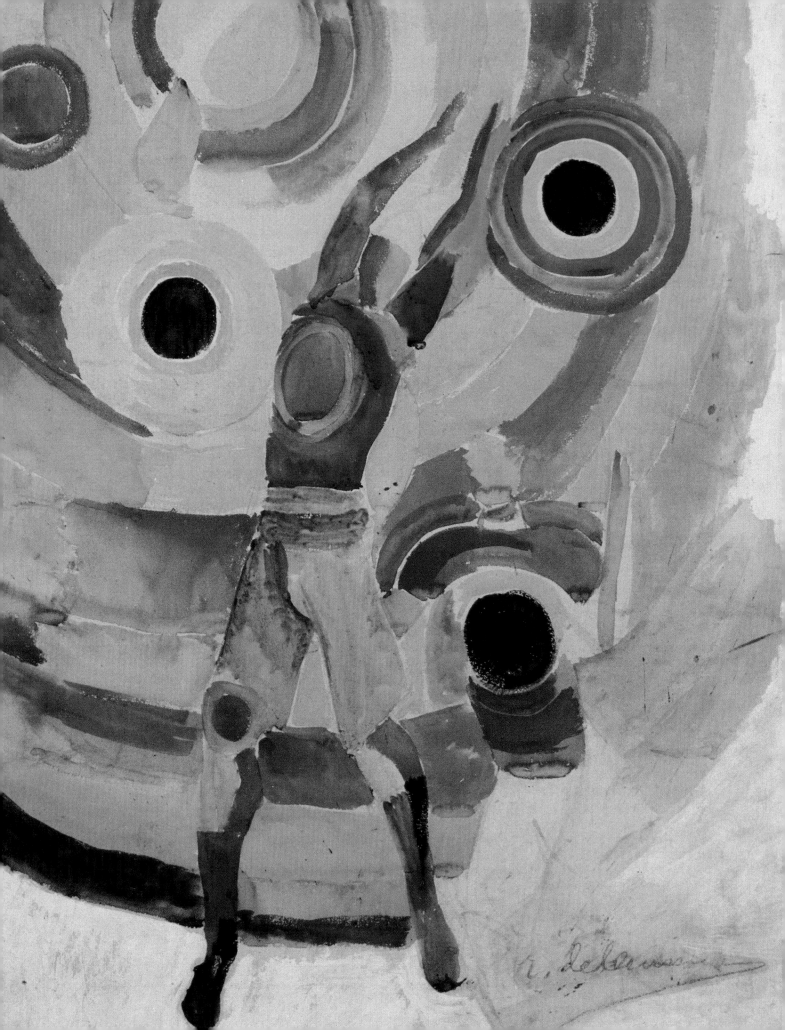

Chapter 7

Breathing Under Pressure

In 1783 the Montgolfier brothers successfully flew their first hot air balloon and made aviation history. For hundreds of years, men had dreamed of emulating the flight of birds, and the twentieth century has seen the attainment and surpassing of many of these dreams, with spectacular advances in aerospace technology.

Man's conquest of the air brought its own problems, however. Atmospheric pressure reduces with increasing altitude, as does the oxygen tension of the air, making it difficult for people to take in sufficient oxygen. While mountain climbers can acclimatize gradually to altitude, allowing their systems time to adapt, sudden exposure to low atmospheric pressure can cause severe distress.

Nearly a hundred years after the Montgolfiers' triumph, in 1875, three young scientists, Crocé-Spinelli, Sivel and Gaston Tissandier, took a balloon to 25,000 feet, but only Tissandier survived; the other two died from respiratory difficulties due to low oxygen levels at reduced atmospheric pressure. Scientists and aviators began to realize that over altitudes of 10,000 feet human beings need to breathe air with an increasing concentration of oxygen until, at 42,000 feet, even 100 percent oxygen at that atmospheric pressure is insufficient to maintain respiration.

If the atmosphere is mechanically pressurized, however, the problem is solved. In a pressurized cabin, air is sucked in and compressed by a motor to maintain the atmosphere at the desired level. In 1931 Auguste Piccard reached a height of 51,762 feet, using a sealed, pressurized cabin beneath his balloon, and Ross and Prather ascended to 113,700 feet by the same means.

At sea level, the atmospheric pressure of air is expressed as being 760 mm Hg, or 760 millimeters of mercury. This means simply that the air will support a column of mercury 760 millimeters high. Oxygen constitutes almost 21 percent of air and thus makes a contribution of just over one-fifth to

The fitter the person, the more efficient are the circulatory systems and the uptake and use of life-giving oxygen. Football *(1917), a vivid, joyous painting by Robert Delaunay, reverberates with the energy of the fit individual who is enjoying life and activity to the full.*

Early planes such as Charles Lindbergh's Spirit of St. Louis, *in which he made the first solo, nonstop transatlantic flight, flew below the heights at which pressurization is necessary.*

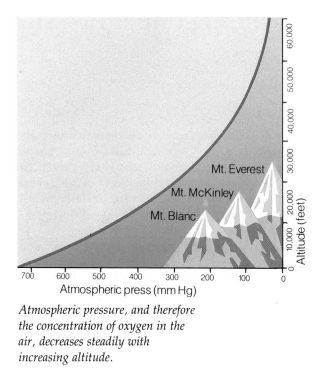

Atmospheric pressure, and therefore the concentration of oxygen in the air, decreases steadily with increasing altitude.

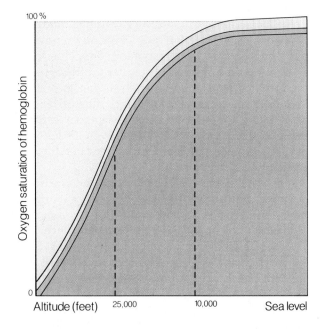

When the oxygen concentration of the air lowers with altitude, the level of saturation of hemoglobin with oxygen is correspondingly reduced.

the 760 mm Hg pressure of the air. Oxygen, then, is said to have a partial pressure of 160 mm Hg (a fifth of the total air pressure).

Altitude and Atmospheric Changes

Both temperature and atmospheric pressure decrease with increasing altitude. At 18,000 feet, atmospheric pressure drops from 760 mm Hg to 380 mm Hg, and the ambient temperature is −20 degrees Centigrade (−4°F). The resulting reduction in the tension, or partial pressure, of oxygen means that the amount of oxygen carried by hemoglobin to the tissues of the body is reduced. The normal concentration of hemoglobin is about 13 grams per 100 milliliters of blood. When 100 percent saturated, as in a healthy individual living at sea level, each gram of hemoglobin can carry 1.34 milliliters of oxygen. Theoretically 100 milliliters of blood can transport 20 milliliters of oxygen to the body tissues. At rest, the heart pumps approximately 5 liters of blood per minute — the cardiac output — so normally, 1,000 milliliters of oxygen are available for use every minute: well in excess of the minimum requirement, while the body is at rest, of 250 milliliters per minute.

The reduction in oxygen tension at altitude is rarely a problem up to 10,000 feet. Beyond this there is such a rapid decline in the oxygen content of hemoglobin that, at 18,000 feet, people unacclimatized to these heights can suffer significant effects from deficiency of oxygen, including faintness and shortness of breath. At 40,000 feet and over, atmospheric pressure is so far reduced that even breathing 100 percent oxygen is insufficient to sustain life.

Modern airplanes generally cruise at 30,000 to 40,000 feet, while Concorde flies at 50,000 to 60,000 feet. At these altitudes, if not protected by pressurized cabins, passengers would be unconscious within fifteen seconds and dead within four minutes. Cabins are pressurized to the equivalent of atmospheric pressure at 6,000 to 8,000 feet instead of to sea level pressure. To do the latter would increase the weight of the airplane and create too great a pressure differential between the inside and outside of the plane. In highly maneuverable combat airplanes, weight can be a crucial factor, and, in order to minimize the load,

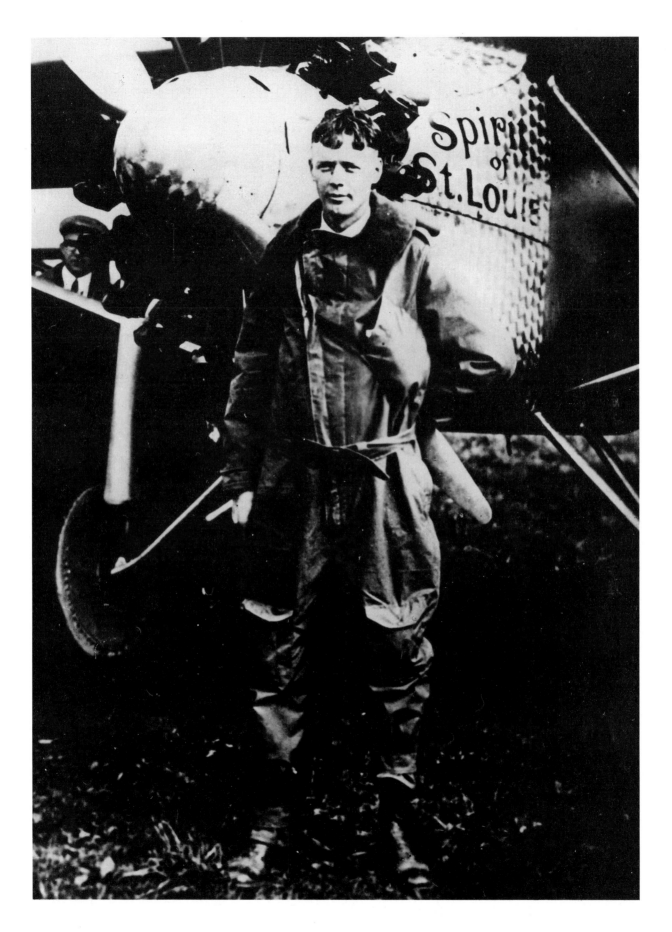

If, in an emergency, cabin pressure in an airplane drops below the equivalent of 14,000 feet, oxygen equipment is automatically released. Scenes of panic as occurred in the movie Airport *are, however, rare.*

Long-term mountain dwellers, such as the Andean Indians, develop changes in the blood, enabling the transport of more oxygen. These changes compensate for the lower oxygen level at high altitude.

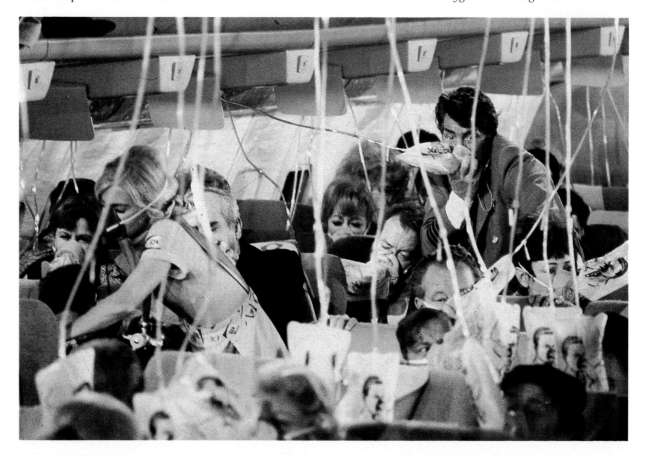

such planes are often unpressurized. The pilot breathes increasing concentrations of oxygen through a mask until at 30,000 feet he receives 100 percent oxygen.

The problems of sudden exposure to low air pressure are best illustrated by the length of time useful consciousness lasts once a person suddenly loses the ground-equivalent oxygen supply. For example, at 21,000 feet useful consciousness remains for ten minutes, at 25,000 feet, for three minutes, at 30,000 feet for one and a quarter minutes and at 60,000 feet for only a quarter of a minute. Thus a pilot whose oxygen supply cuts out at 30,000 feet has only just over a minute to descend to an altitude at which oxygen tension is sufficient to prevent loss of consciousness.

Characteristics of lower-than-normal levels of oxygen in the blood at altitude vary from person to person and can depend, in mountain climbers for example, on the rate of ascent. People may experience subtle personality changes, euphoria, loss of judgment and short-term memory, poor performance and mental coordination, and slurred speech. These changes could cause a pilot to crash his airplane or a mountaineer to continue his ascent without oxygen.

Sudden exposure to low oxygen levels makes the body try to compensate by increasing the heart rate and cardiac output in order to maintain oxygen supply to the tissues. The oxygen level may be low enough to stimulate chemoreceptors to increase the rate of respiration.

While pilots and airplane passengers must be protected by pressurized surroundings in order not to be exposed suddenly to low atmospheric pressure, mountaineers and mountain dwellers gradually adapt to their surroundings. In Peru, about four and a half million people live in the Andes at altitudes of over 10,000 feet; more than 160,000 live in mining villages at over 14,000 feet

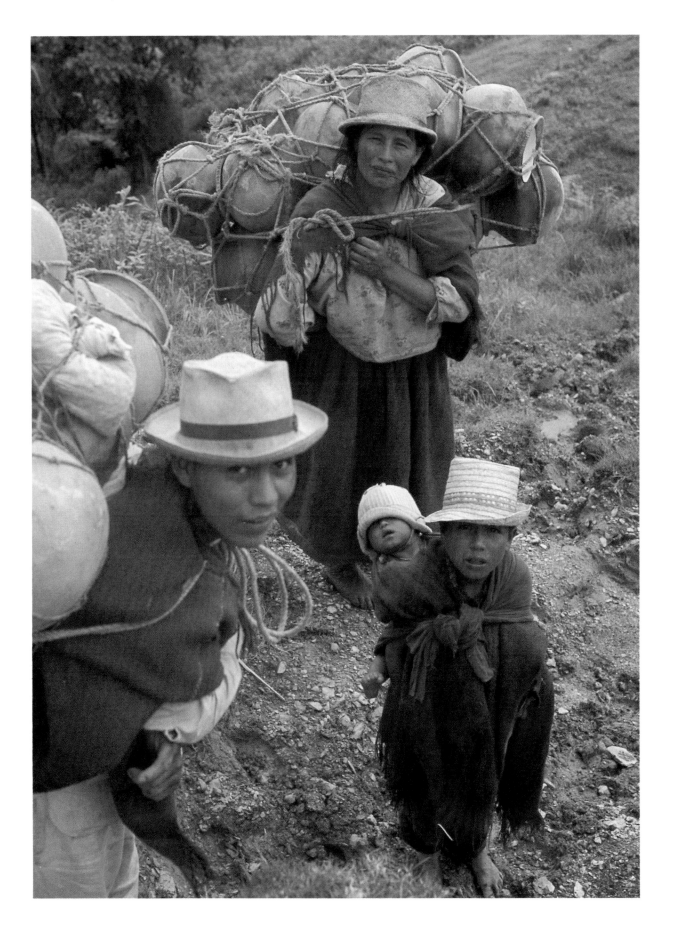

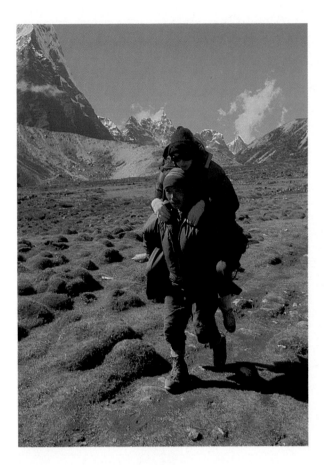

Without sufficient acclimatization, people unused to high altitude risk severe ill-effects. A Sherpa carries a trekker suffering from acute mountain sickness (above) *down to a hospital at 14,000 feet, proving the point that he, born and bred in the Himalayas, is perfectly at ease in conditions which have induced severe illness in the lowlander.*

and work still higher, in mines above 16,000 feet. These people and other long-term mountain dwellers develop changes in the blood enabling more oxygen to be carried.

Research carried out on the Sherpas of the Himalayas, people born and bred in the mountains, shows that they respond much less to the low oxygen conditions at altitude and cope better with the low oxygen levels than do lowlanders who have simply become well acclimatized. In the long-term residents there are fundamental adaptations, perhaps at a cellular level, allowing them to function efficiently at altitude. It is not known to what extent these adjustments are genetic in origin.

Acclimatizing to Altitude

A lowlander merely undergoes a series of gradual short-term adjustments allowing survival in conditions of low oxygen tension at altitude. For successful acclimatization, time must be spent at progressively higher altitudes, allowing the respiratory processes to make the necessary changes. Mountain climbers must ascend slowly, making regular stops at base camps to allow their bodies time to adjust to the new conditions. In theory, they can reach 21,000 feet comfortably in this way but above this should carry oxygen equipment as a safeguard. There are several ways in which the body adjusts to cope with altitude.

At high altitudes, ventilation is usually no longer controlled by the carbon dioxide concentration in the blood but by the stimulation of low oxygen levels — the so-called hypoxic drive. By hyperventilating — taking numerous deep breaths in rapid succession — more carbon dioxide is blown off from the body, allowing room for higher oxygen tension in the alveoli. It is possible for a climber to reach the top of Everest without oxygen equipment partly by means of hyperventilation.

After adequate acclimatization, the hemoglobin releases oxygen to the tissues more readily, thus helping to ensure adequate oxygenation. This is the result of an actual alteration in the hemoglobin molecule in response to the low oxygen tension in the body. Yet another response of the body is the release of a substance known as erythropoietin, from the kidney, that stimulates the bone marrow to produce more red blood cells. The increase in

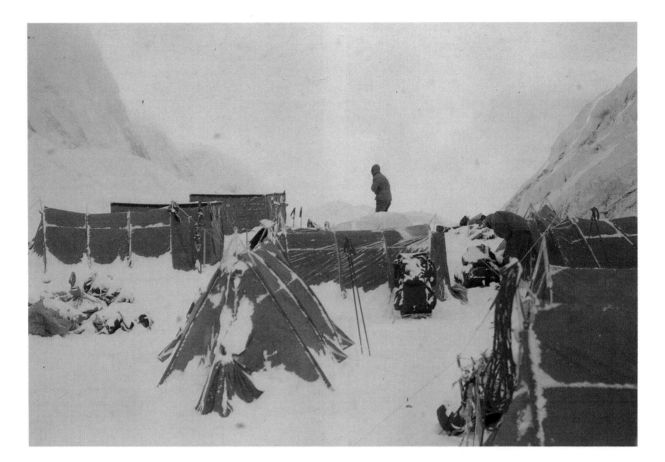

hemoglobin available to carry oxygen, and consequent greater oxygen-carrying capabilities of the blood, offset the reduction in oxygen tension. Residents at high altitudes have a higher hemoglobin level per 100 milliliters of blood than people at sea level. A third result of acclimatization is that new capillaries appear and maintain the delivery of oxygen to the tissues.

Mountain Sickness

Mountain sickness is the mountain climber's equivalent of the diver's decompression sickness — both essentially physical problems caused by pressure changes. In its milder forms, it causes headache, fatigue, dizziness, palpitations, loss of appetite, nausea and insomnia. The condition was described as early as 326 B.C. by Plutarch in his account of Alexander the Great crossing the mountains into India. In A.D. 100 a Chinese writer took mountain sickness as a sign that the natural

Mountaineers taking part in trips such as the International Everest Expedition need time for proper acclimatization to altitude and undergo a period of training and exercise at progressively higher levels. During ascent, they must make regular stops at base camps to allow their bodies time to adjust to conditions. This Everest camp is pictured after a heavy snow storm.

The low oxygen conditions near the
summit of Everest are such that the
human body operates at the very
limits of its tolerance. Climbers have
made the ascent without the use of
supplementary oxygen, however.

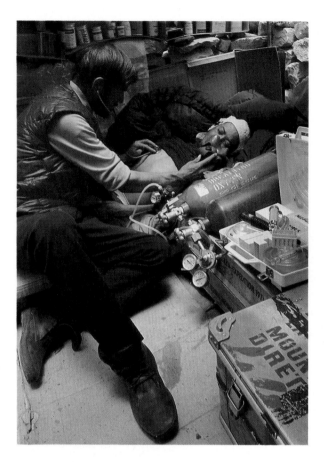

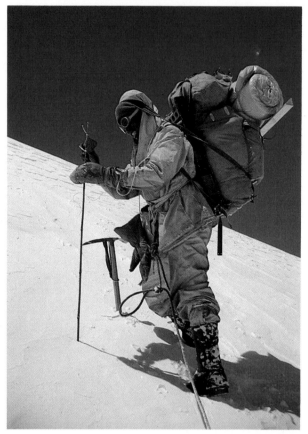

*A climber, suffering from high
altitude pulmonary edema, is treated
with oxygen at a base camp hospital,
until he can be transferred to lower
altitude. In this acute condition,
fluid fills the lung alveoli and
prevents normal gas exchange.*

boundaries of China should not be crossed,
describing the "greater and lesser headache
mountains." The Spanish *conquistadors* noted that
their livestock became less fertile at high altitudes in
the Andes, and this realization may have encouraged the transfer of the capital of Peru from an
altitude of 10,900 feet to Lima at a mere 500 feet.

The more severe forms of mountain sickness can
be fatal for a person suddenly removed to high
altitude. In the condition known as high altitude
pulmonary edema, or HAPE, the lung alveoli fill up
with fluid; liquid from the blood plasma passes
from the alveolar capillaries into the air spaces,
severely impairing gas exchange. The reasons for
the onset of this condition are not clear but may be
related to a rise in pressure in the pulmonary blood
vessels. The balance within the pulmonary system
is thus disturbed and fluid is pushed out from the
vessels into the alveoli. HAPE can be prevented by
slow ascent, allowing time for acclimatization, and

*With the prospect of astronauts
spending longer and longer in space
in Spacelab and orbiting space
stations, NASA experiments are
underway to assess the effects of
weightlessness on lung function.*

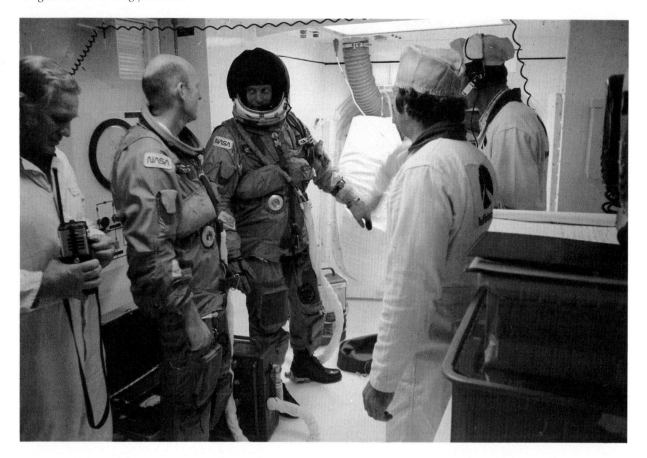

many climbers take a drug, acetazolamide, which behaves as a diuretic, increasing urinary excretion of sodium and water. This appears to reduce the risk of pulmonary edema.

A person suffering from HAPE must be taken to a lower altitude as soon as possible, meanwhile receiving oxygen and diuretic therapy. Even residents of high altitudes can suffer HAPE. In one such case, a man returning to his own village after a two-week visit to relatives at sea level developed pulmonary edema.

Even the body's own efforts to combat the stresses of altitude can have side effects. The response to produce more red blood cells to improve oxygenation increases the viscosity of the blood and hence the likelihood of clots forming within blood vessels. People living at 15,000 feet have hemoglobin concentrations of half as much again as the normal level, and there is an increased incidence of strokes among these people.

Space travel takes mankind to undreamed of distances from Earth. For more than two decades, human beings have been traveling into space, some surviving there for as long as six months. There are three major problems space travelers must contend with: first, solar radiation, since they are no longer protected by the Earth's atmosphere; second, the effect of acceleration and deceleration on leaving and reentering the Earth's atmosphere; and third, the effects of the absence of atmospheric pressure and gravity. The latter two have direct effects on respiration.

The Stresses of Space Travel

To leave the Earth's atmosphere and escape its gravitational field, a spacecraft must attain a speed of about 25,000 miles an hour, requiring high acceleration rates. The so-called g-forces of rapid acceleration at launching and deceleration during reentry impose marked stress forces on the tissues

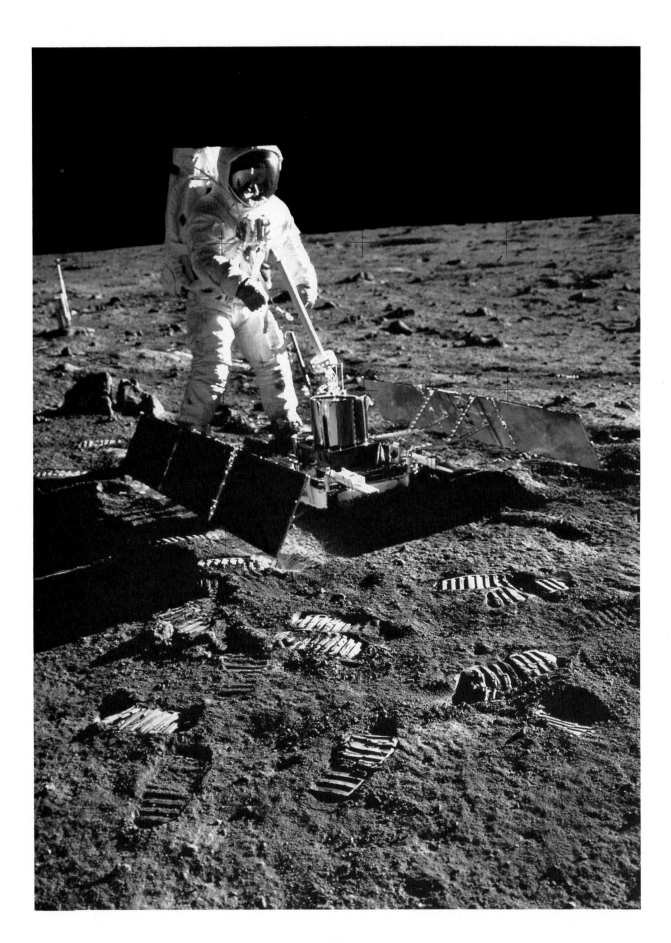

Since there is no atmosphere on the moon, astronauts must carry their own breathing mix. During his lunar walk, Apollo crew member Aldrin breathed 100 percent oxygen at a lower than atmospheric pressure.

of the body and, theoretically, can create tearing forces between mobile and immobile tissues. The effect on the lungs and chest of this degree of acceleration is to cause two liters of blood and interstitial fluid to leave the legs and redistribute to the thorax and head, giving the astronaut a puffy face and overdistended neck veins. It is estimated that the volume of fluid in the legs alters by about 13 percent during acceleration. To offset the effects of g-forces, astronauts should lie down during take off and reentry and wear special antigravity suits. On acceleration, these suits automatically pump up, and the increased pressure they put on the body prevents pooling of the blood.

If the astronaut remains in an erect position, blood distribution in the lungs alters dramatically, blood leaving the top of the lung in preference for the lung bases. The normal difference in intrapleural pressure between the top and bottom of the lung is increased dramatically, and this increase is responsible for a marked exaggeration of mismatching between ventilation and blood flow in the lungs. At the top of the lungs, alveolar ventilation may be perfect, but perfusion may be zero — equivalent essentially to increasing the dead space of the respiratory tract and lungs. At the lung bases, there may be so much venous congestion and edema, due to the relative increase in blood flow, that airways and alveoli start to close off, and circulation takes place without ventilation.

At up to six times gravity (6 g), the respiratory muscles have sufficient strength to lift the rib cage, which becomes increasingly heavy due to gravity, and to move the diaphragm and attached abdominal viscera. The respiratory rate usually increases, and the tidal volume decreases in response to the over-distended upper and collapsed lower lungs.

Redistribution of blood from the legs to the thorax causes the heart to increase its rate and output. There is also an altered pattern of salt and water excretion by the kidneys.

Once in orbit, man becomes weightless. Even after twelve days on the Apollo missions, astronauts showed an 8 percent reduction in plasma volume and a 10 percent reduction in red blood cells. The effect of weightlessness on the lungs is to minimize the mismatch between ventilation and blood flow and make the two more

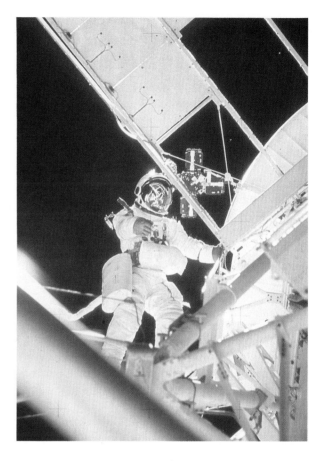

An astronaut performing extravehicular activities in space is stretching his physical capabilities to the utmost to withstand the stresses of extreme temperatures, zero gravity and atmosphere, and weightlessness. His spacesuit provides a controlled mini-environment, but the long-term effects of such hazards on man's physiology are yet to be understood.

uniform than they are on Earth. Theoretically, gas exchange should improve, and astronauts seem to show no decrease in their work capacity while weightless.

On return to Earth, however, both work capacity and cardiac output are below normal; even sitting up may cause low blood pressure because of the reduction in plasma volume. Despite vigorous inflight exercise programs and dietary manipulation, muscle mass may decrease in astronauts and bone calcium levels reduce by 4 grams per month while they are in space. Even five years after returning from a space flight, astronauts have been found to have decreased levels of mineral content in their bones.

Since there is no atmosphere in space, the astronauts are provided with one. The spacecraft must be pressurized and equipped with suitable supplies of air. The Russian space program tends to use 21 percent of oxygen in nitrogen at a pressure equivalent to sea level on Earth (one atmosphere), while the Apollo missions used 100 percent oxygen at one-third of an atmosphere. Yet another possible combination is to use 50 percent oxygen at one-half of an atmosphere.

The type of atmospheric condition chosen depends on the weight and space available — using one atmosphere gives a greater weight load than one-third of an atmosphere. Breathing 100 percent oxygen at atmospheric pressure can cause oxygen toxicity, which manifests itself by pulmonary edema, lung fibrosis and convulsions. However, these problems do not occur with pure oxygen used at lower than normal pressures.

Alveolar atelectasis is another problem related to breathing 100 percent oxygen. In the absence of an inert gas, such as nitrogen, if the alveolus becomes temporarily blocked by a plug of sputum, the pressure gradient between alveolus and blood is so steep that the alveolus will collapse. When nitrogen is present in the atmosphere being breathed, this collapse does not occur because the nitrogen keeps the alveolus open until the blockage is cleared. Surface tension forces are such that, once collapsed, the alveoli are extremely difficult to reopen. In this situation, there may be such a significant decrease in lung volume and increase in shunting that, although 100 percent oxygen is being

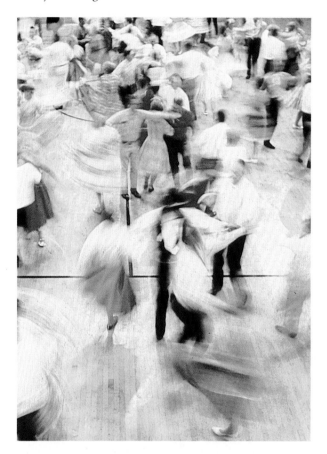

breathed, the blood may be less well oxygenated than when air is breathed.

The Effects of Exercise

Ventilation increases in response to muscular exercise. Exactly why is still not clear, despite the fact that most respiratory physiologists of the last hundred years have studied the association.

When the body is at rest, the oxygen requirement of the tissues is about a quarter of a liter a minute. During exercise this requirement may increase to 4 liters a minute. To ensure that enough oxygen reaches the tissues, cardiac output may increase from 4 to 35 liters of blood a minute, and the volume of respiration (respiratory rate times the amount of air moved in each breath) may increase to over 120 liters of air a minute. Thus the lungs are inflating more rapidly and taking in more air, and, at the same time, there is a large increase in blood flow. While blood flow increases to both upper and lower

Participants in this bicycle race in nineteenth-century Paris are taking aerobic exercise. Like swimming and running, cycling makes the body work harder to provide the oxygen the muscles demand.

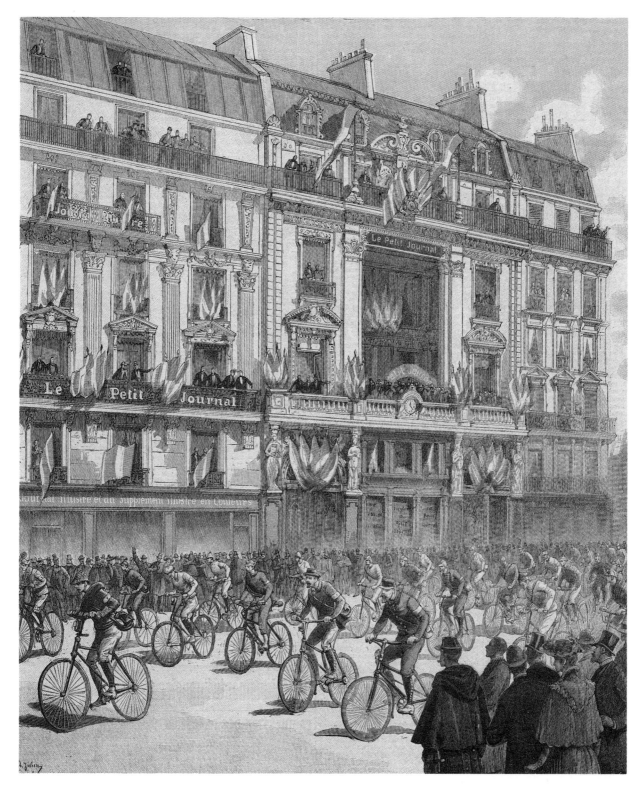

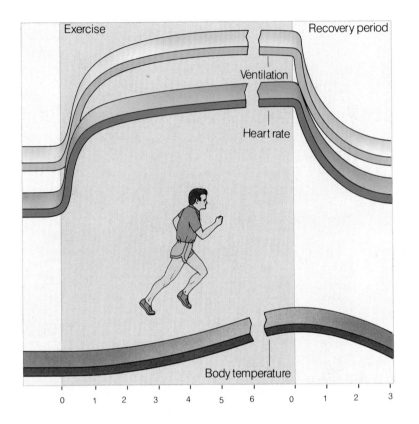

Exercise   Recovery period

Ventilation

Heart rate

Body temperature

0 1 2 3 4 5 6 0 1 2 3

When a person takes vigorous exercise, there is an abrupt increase in ventilation at the onset of activity and an equally sudden drop at the end. Heart rate, too, increases and both ventilation and heart rate eventually reach a plateau. Body temperature also rises with exercise but less dramatically.

zones of the lungs, the increase is greater to the upper zone. As a result, the blood flow to the lungs is more uniform than when the body is at rest.

Energy for exercise is normally obtained from "aerobic" metabolism. In this process, glucose enters cells and is metabolized to pyruvic acid, which then itself enters a series of metabolic changes known as the Krebs cycle. The operation of these changes requires oxygen, and one molecule of glucose can generate 36 molecules of adenosine triphosphate or ATP — the molecule that provides energy for all the metabolic processes in the body. Aerobic exercise requires plenty of oxygen to fuel the body processes and makes us breathe harder to provide it. Aerobic means "with oxygen."

Anaerobic exercise is activity performed in short, high-energy bursts — sprinting for example — or simply activity performed with insufficient oxygen available. There is not time for the oxygen needs to be met, so energy is produced without it; anaerobic

means "without oxygen." In this form of exercise, instead of entering the Krebs cycle, pyruvic acid is converted to lactic acid and only two molecules of ATP are generated per molecule of glucose. When the body is at rest again, the lactic acid can be reconverted to pyruvic acid.

The anaerobic metabolism is inefficient and self-limiting because so much acid is built up that the metabolism is inhibited. At the end of the exercise, breathing does not immediately return to normal but stays at an increased level to repay the oxygen debt. During this time the lactic acid built up can be metabolized.

The answer to the question of why ventilation increases with exercise is still unknown, but there have been several theories. The increase occurs abruptly with the beginning, and terminates abruptly at the end, of exercise. One idea is that the stimulus to increase ventilation comes from the increased carbon dioxide produced by muscular

In a short burst of high speed activity, such as a sprint, there is not enough time for the respiratory system to meet the body's increased oxygen demands. Energy is, therefore, produced anaerobically — without oxygen. At the end of the sprint, the runner's breathing will remain at an increased rate until the body's oxygen level is restored. Sports such as tennis and squash also depend on anaerobic energy.

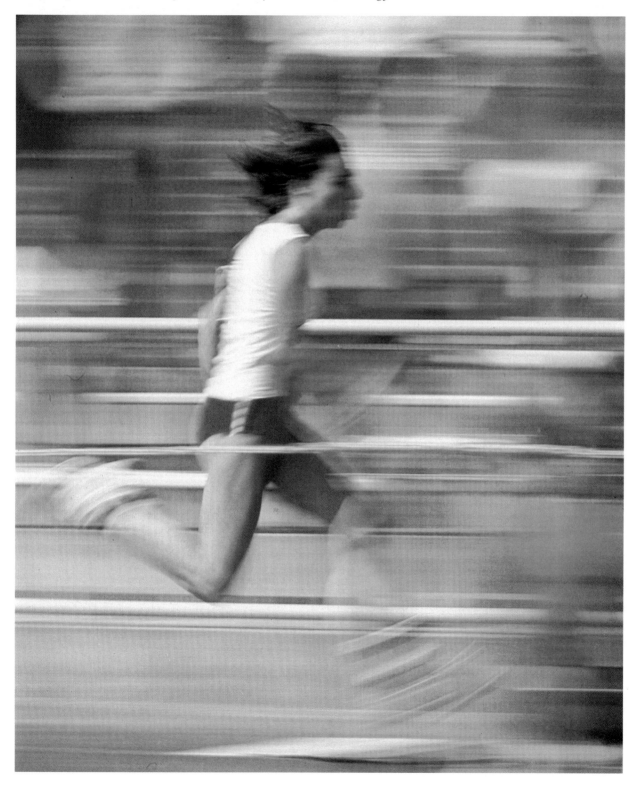

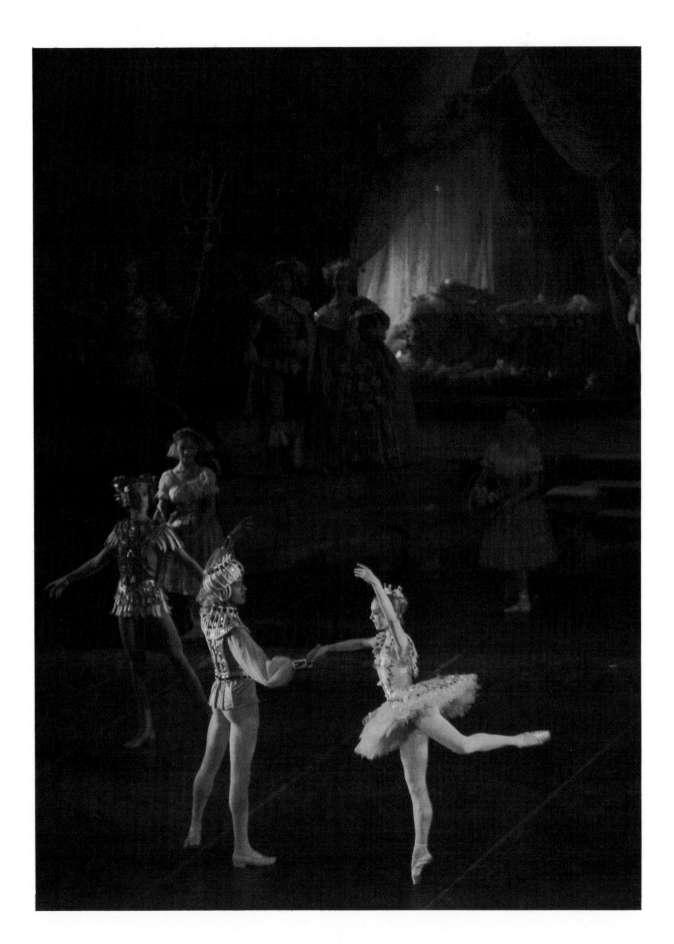

The timing and control of breathing play an essential part in ballet. The dancer learns to seize opportunities to breathe and to coordinate in and out breaths with appropriate movements.

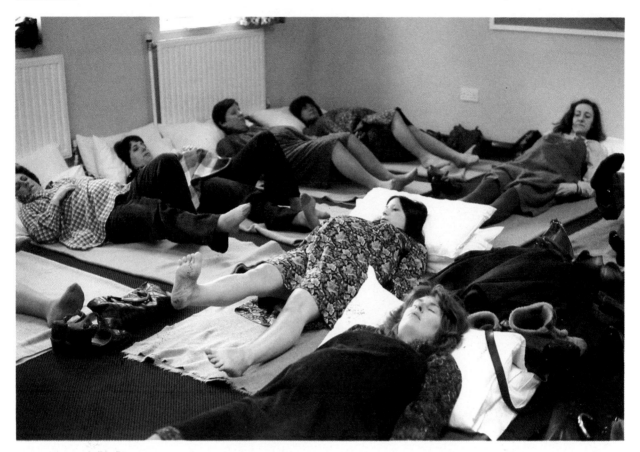

activity, but there is little evidence to support this. The increase occurs before the increase of carbon dioxide tension in the blood could be possible, and, what is more, minute volume (the amount of air moved each minute) may increase fifteen times without any increase in the carbon dioxide tension.

Another theory is that a decrease in oxygen explains the exercise-induced increase in ventilation. More oxygen is consumed during exercise, so it follows that the oxygen tension in the blood decreases unless ventilation is increased. However, reduced oxygen tension is not usual in anything other than extremely vigorous exercise; in fact, a slight rise in tension is more common. Many other reasons for the stimulus have been put forward, including the alteration of the acid-alkali, or pH, balance in the blood and rise in temperature, but there are now two more likely explanations.

First, that the increase occurs as a response to simultaneous impulses from the brain going both to

Correct breathing can be of great benefit during childbirth, and many expectant mothers attend classes to practice breathing for labor. Deep, calming breaths help the body relax in the early stages, whereas tension and holding the breath increase pain. At classes, mothers also learn how gentle, panting breaths can help them through contractions.

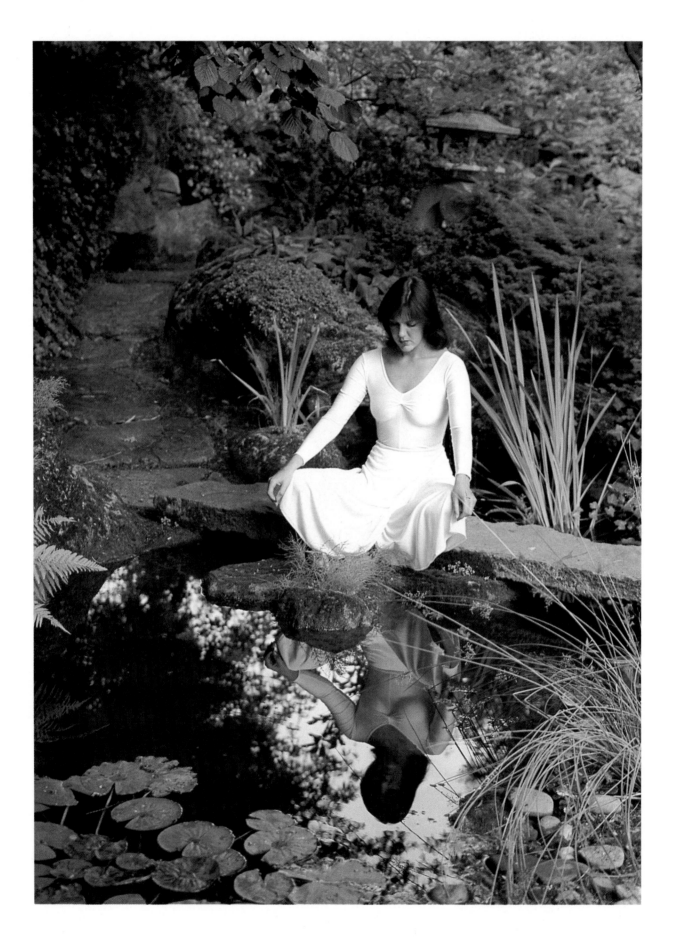

Breathing exercises, often practiced while seated in the lotus position (left), are an essential part of yoga; they are helpful in attaining the breathing control necessary to achieve and sustain yoga postures.

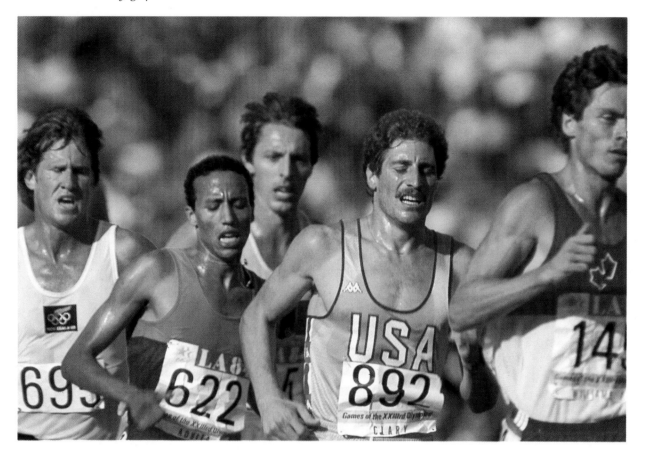

the muscles that will increase their activity on exercise and to the muscles involved in respiration. Second, that movements in the limbs immediately stimulate joint receptors, which relay back messages to the brain to increase ventilation. The fact that passive limb movements — a person's limbs being moved by someone else or mechanically — are followed by an increase in ventilation would seem to support the latter theory.

In certain conditions, breathing problems may follow exercise. A person performing vigorous exercise at high altitude, for example, may suffer hypoxemia — low oxygen in the bloodstream — because the oxygen he is taking in is inadequate to fuel his activity. Extreme activity in conditions of atmospheric pollution can also cause post-exercise problems. At the 1984 Los Angeles Olympics, there was controversy about athletes being required to perform in an environment polluted by industrial and automobile fumes. Particular conditions in Los

Competitors in long and middle distance track events have a high and efficient level of oxygen consumption. Sustained training in aerobic activity, such as running, cycling or swimming, increases the body's oxygen consumption and its ability to make use of that oxygen, thus improving overall fitness.

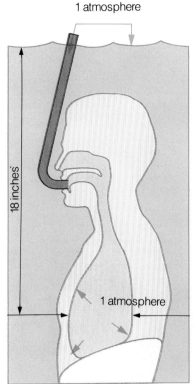

1 atmosphere

18 inches

1 atmosphere

1 atmosphere + 18 inches of water

At depths down to 18 inches of water, a human being can breathe through a snorkel — a tube through which air passes from the surface to the mouth. Below this level, even with a longer tube, breathing through a snorkel is impossible for two reasons. First, air would simply be moved up and down the tube, and no new air would enter the lungs. Second, the diver would be unable to expand his chest, filled with air at sea level pressure, against the water surrounding it at greater than sea level pressure.

Angeles cause hot air to be trapped by cold air higher up instead of rising and dispersing, so pollutants take a long time to escape to the upper atmosphere.

A High Pressure Environment

While decreasing atmospheric pressure makes breathing difficult at high altitude, diving underwater can cause respiratory problems because of greatly increased pressure. At the water surface, the pressure is one atmosphere; 33 feet of water also exerts the pressure equivalent of one atmosphere, so at this depth a diver is subject to a pressure of two atmospheres. With every 33 feet of additional depth, the pressure increases one atmosphere.

Underwater, a human being must either hold his breath until returning to the surface or breathe through some sort of equipment. Down to about 18 inches, all that is necessary is a snorkel — an open tube to the surface. Below this, however long the tube provided, the diver is unable to expand his chest, filled with air at sea level atmospheric pressure, against the water now surrounding his chest at much greater pressure. Moreover, even if he did manage to move his chest, he would simply be moving air up and down the tube, which would in effect become an extension of the dead space formed by the upper airways. There would be no exchange of air, and carbon dioxide would build up in the body.

Without special equipment, a human diver can only descend deeper than 18 inches by a breath-holding dive. The danger is that, while the diver is holding his breath, carbon dioxide is building up to the level which should stimulate another breath. If the diver fails to resume breathing in time, he can become unconscious underwater, due to lack of oxygen in the bloodstream, and drown. Although even an experienced diver finds it difficult to descend below 33 feet, the world record for a breath-holding dive is reputed to be an astounding 280 feet.

Throughout history, man has attempted to make equipment to allow divers to remain underwater for longer periods. One early invention was the diving bell, a container in which the diver stood and was then lowered into the water. He breathed the air present in the bell at the time of submersion.

In scuba diving — SCUBA stands for Self-contained Underwater Breathing Apparatus — the diver is supplied with compressed air at ambient pressure from a tank he carries on his back.

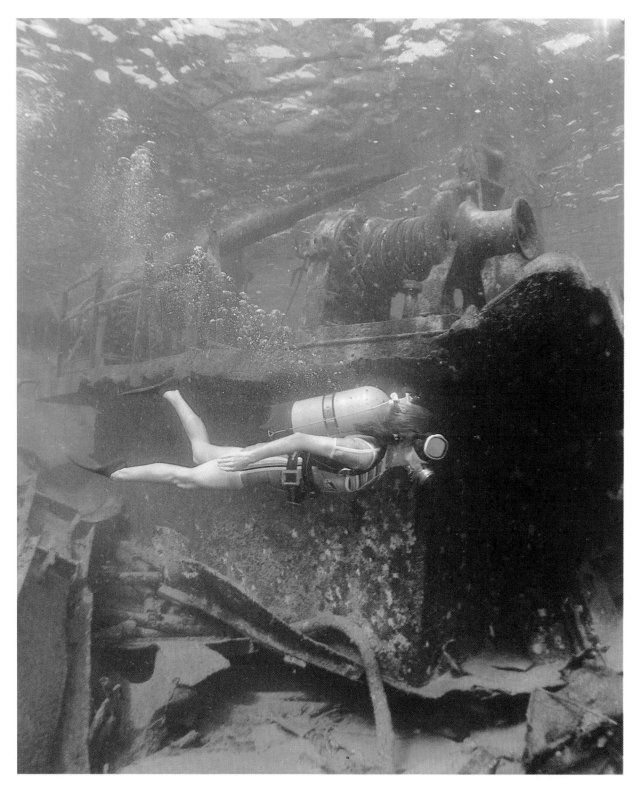

In the earliest diving bells, the only
air available to the diver was that
present in the bell at submersion.
Diving suits first appeared in the
1700s, the wearer breathing air
pumped from the surface.

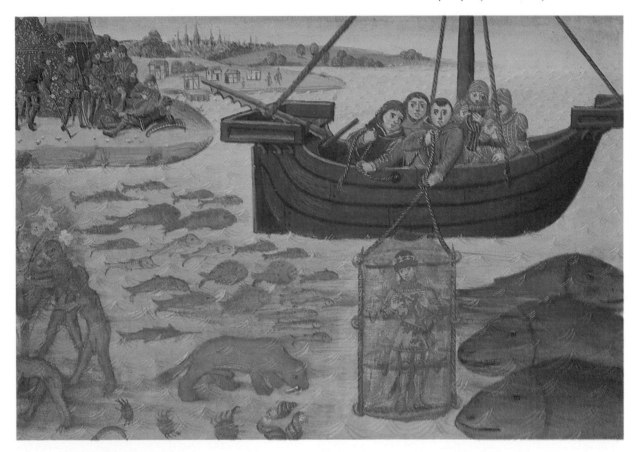

*As early as the fourth century B.C.
Alexander the Great is said to have
descended below the surface of the
Mediterranean Sea in a structure
resembling a diving bell. From this
he was able to observe underwater
creatures. An imaginative variety of
marine life is depicted in this version
of his exploits.*

Following the development of the diving helmet
early in the nineteenth century, Auguste Siebe, in
1837, produced the first enclosed diving suit, which
remained essentially unchanged for the next
hundred years. The diver wore a metal helmet and
watertight suit and was supplied with air through
lines from the surface. Nowadays, in such systems,
the heavy metal helmet has been replaced by lighter
fiber glass.

In the 1940s, SCUBA equipment (Self-contained
Underwater Breathing Apparatus) was first tested.
The diver wears a light, waterproof suit and carries
air cylinders on his back, thus freeing him from the
surface. He breathes gas from the cylinders at a
pressure equal to that exerted on his chest by the
particular depth of water. The diver is safe on
descent and while at depth, but must observe
certain precautions on ascent. If he holds his breath
on ascent, the tension of the air in his lungs
increases while the pressure outside on his chest is

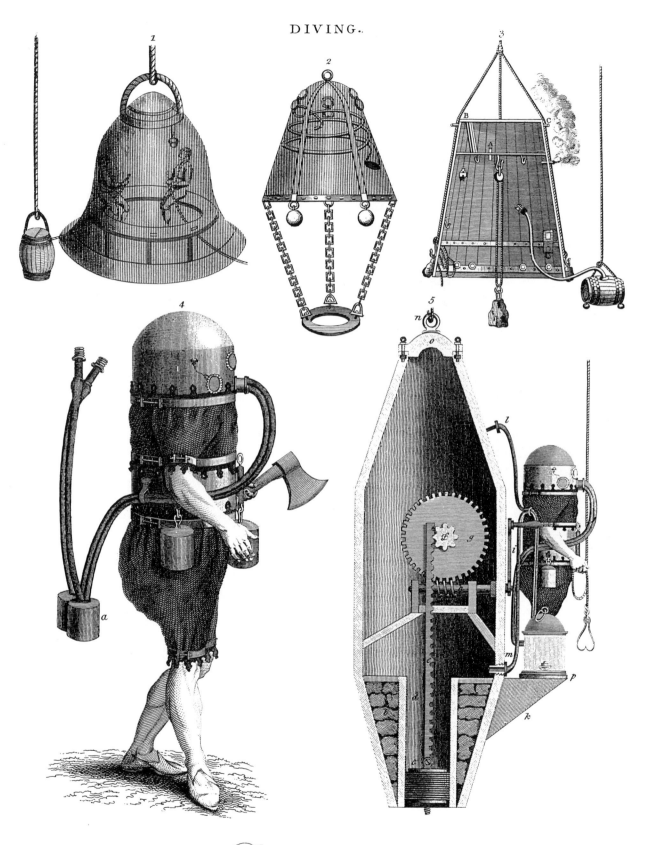

Diving Machines.

J. Pass sculp.

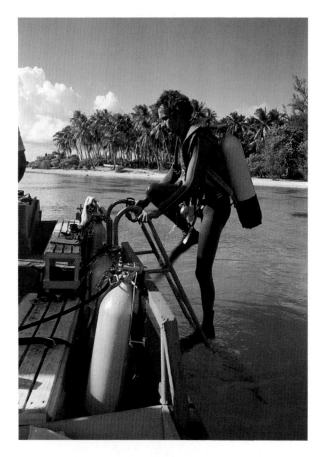

A valve on the scuba tank supplies air as the diver's breathing demands. Down to between 100 and 165 feet, compressed air can be used to fill the tank, but, below this, the nitrogen contained in air becomes narcotic, and a mixture of oxygen and helium is considered safer.

decreasing; the alveoli and airways swell and can rupture. Bubbles of air can pass from the alveoli to the blood vessels and enter the circulation, blocking vessels and cutting off blood supply to parts of the body. Divers must be trained to breathe normally during a slow ascent or to exhale vigorously during a rapid ascent.

The mixture of gas supplied to the diver, by whatever means, varies according to depth. Pure oxygen cannot be used at depths greater than 25 feet since, at pressure, 100 percent oxygen is toxic and can cause oxygen poisoning and convulsions. Below 25 feet, compressed air is used. But, below 100 feet, the pressure of nitrogen also increases rapidly. Nitrogen concentration builds up in the body and the tissues absorb the gas.

The "Bends"

While the diver may descend as fast as he likes, it is the ascent that can cause problems when breathing gas containing nitrogen. As he ascends, nitrogen is released from the tissues; and if the ascent is slow, the circulation collects the nitrogen and releases it through the respiratory system. If the ascent is too rapid, however, nitrogen may bubble out of the blood and collect in tissues — particularly those around the joints — causing the syndrome known as the "bends." The automatic response to the pain of this condition is to bend the affected joints in an attempt to ease the pain — hence the name. In its mild form, the bends may cause pain in the joints, itching and fatigue, while a more serious case may involve giddiness, paralysis and severe respiratory distress.

Paul Bert, in his book published in 1878, showed that decompression sickness was due to a release of nitrogen into the blood and tissues. The only effective treatment for the condition is recompression under medical supervision. In the recompression chamber, the air bubbles in the diver's body gradually disperse; he or she is then slowly brought back to atmospheric pressure.

The risk of decompression sickness increases both with the depth reached and the amount of time spent at that depth. Commercial divers, who may spend prolonged periods working at extreme depth on oil rigs or pipe lines, are particularly at risk and, on return to the surface, must stay in a

Paul Bert

The Founder of Aerospace Medicine

The first aeronaut casualties were two French balloonists, Sivel and Crocé-Spinelli. Together with Gaston Tissandier, they began their ascent on April 15, 1875 with a far from adequate supply of oxygen, despite warnings from their friend Paul Bert, the pioneer of high altitude physiology. On reaching 26,000 feet the balloonists found they were too weak to breathe. Miraculously, Tissandier survived, but the other two perished, suffering from respiratory failure.

All France was shocked, none more so than Paul Bert who had worked for years on the effects of abnormal pressures on the human body. Born in 1833, in Auxerre, France. Bert first became a lawyer before studying medicine and natural sciences in Paris. After receiving an MD in 1863, he studied under the famous physiologist Claude Bernard at the Collège de France, and, in 1869, succeeded Bernard to the Chair of Physiology at the Sorbonne in Paris, where he remained until 1886.

While at the Sorbonne, Bert made a systematic study of the decompression sickness suffered by divers. Known later as "the bends," this ailment was shown by Bert to be the result of surfacing too quickly from regions of high pressure. He demonstrated how, under high

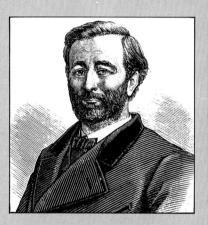

pressures, gases dissolve in the blood and body tissues. He also showed how very rapid decompression causes nitrogen in particular, to bubble out of the tissues, obstructing the capillaries and resulting in possibly fatal cramps. As a preventative, he developed the successful method of slow, gradual decompression still in use today.

The first man to study the behavior of blood under a range of gas pressures, Bert came to the fundamental conclusion that the physiological effects of oxygen in the blood are due to its partial pressure, regardless of atmospheric pressure or the amount of oxygen. "Oxygen tension is everything," he wrote, "barometric pressure in itself is nothing or almost nothing."

To investigate the physiological effects of high altitude, Bert built himself a steel decompression chamber, large

enough to hold a human being. After experimenting on himself and on animals, he concluded that it was the reduced partial pressure of oxygen — in the air breathed, in the blood and in the tissues — that caused the damaging consequences of high altitudes. He found that these effects could be avoided by breathing supplementary oxygen.

In 1878, Bert published his work in a book, *La Pression Barometrique*, which has become a classic in physiology since its translation into English in 1943. The theories put forward in this book were of great importance in aviation medicine during World War II. Bert has been called the founder of aerospace medicine, but his pioneering research has helped to make possible the exploration not only of space but also of the ocean depths.

For the last fifteen years of his life, Bert was involved in politics. Elected to the Chamber of Deputies in 1872 and made Education Minister, he was responsible for major changes in both elementary and higher education. He was also a great popularizer of science and published many school text books on the natural sciences. In 1886, he was appointed Governor-General of French Indo-China, where he died of dysentery only a few months after his arrival.

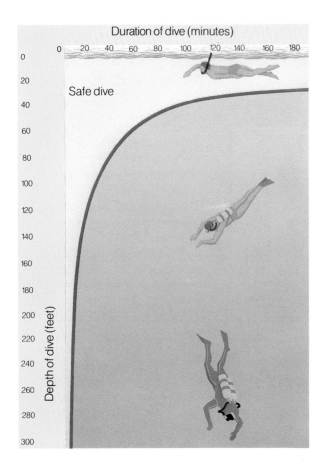

Duration of dive (minutes)

Safe dive

Depth of dive (feet)

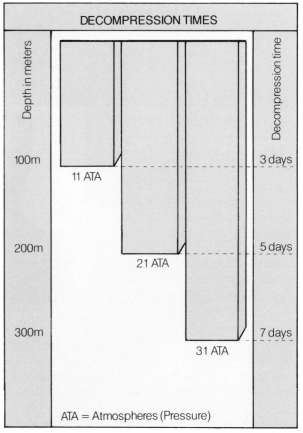

DECOMPRESSION TIMES

Depth in meters

Decompression time

100m — 11 ATA — 3 days

200m — 21 ATA — 5 days

300m — 31 ATA — 7 days

ATA = Atmospheres (Pressure)

The deeper the dive, the shorter should be its duration if the diver is to surface directly without risk of decompression sickness. The shallower the dive, the longer the diver may remain under safely. Times and depths of safe dives are published by diving organizations (above). Commercial divers may have to spend prolonged periods at great depths, necessitating gradual recovery in a pressure chamber. Typical decompression times are shown in the chart (above right).

pressure chamber on their boat or rig while they decompress over several days.

Below about 165 feet, nitrogen becomes increasingly narcotic, and divers descending to great depths generally use a mixture of oxygen and helium. Helium is less soluble in body fat so is less likely to be stored and form bubbles. Its small molecular size allows it to diffuse more rapidly than nitrogen, aiding decompression.

Much of the current research into underwater technology is concerned with reducing the time for decompression without increasing the incidence of decompression sickness. With the exploration and exploitation of oceanic oilfields and other resources of the seabed, such considerations have become commercially important. In the meantime, however, all divers, amateur and commercial, must make a careful study of the advised limits of the depth, duration and frequency of dives. It is also unwise to fly within 24 hours of diving. The

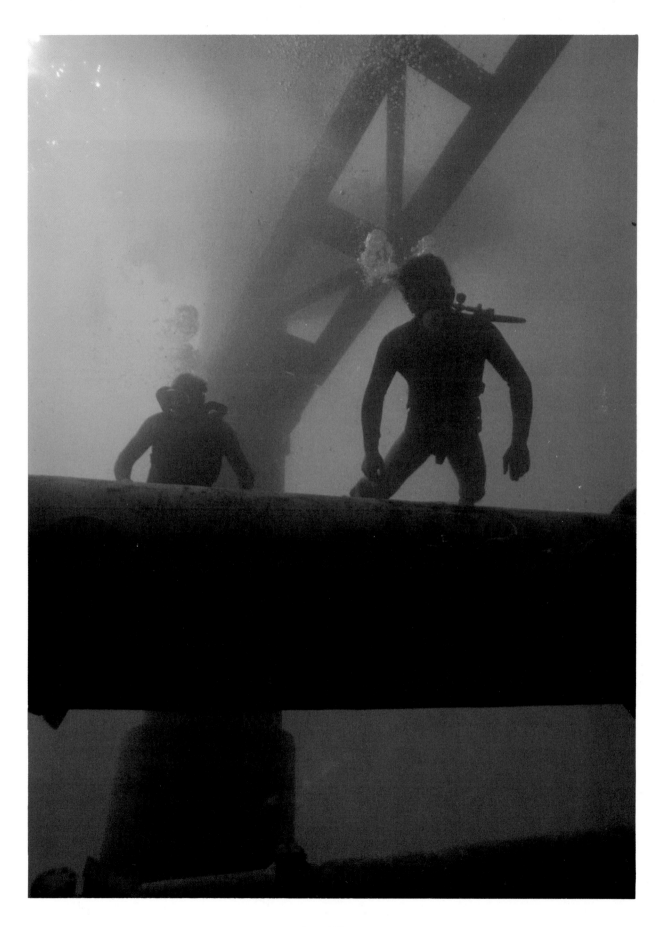

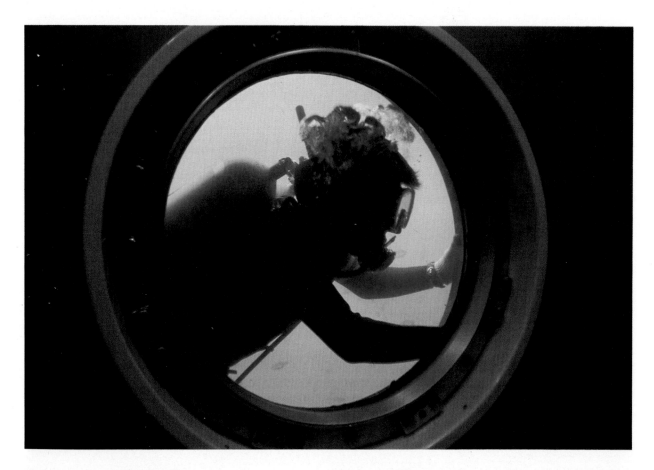

Underwater towers, from which divers can observe the marine world in safety, have stimulated interest and research in long-term underwater habitats. Such pressure-proof environments, in which people can work and live, are of great importance for industries such as offshore oil rigs.

pressure difference between the deep sea and the aircraft can cause the traveler to suffer the "bends."

Underwater Man

The possibility of man adapting anatomically to survival at depth has long intrigued the world, and submarines, submersibles and sealabs are all attempts to allow humans to remain and work underwater for long periods. In 1963, marine biologist Jacques Cousteau described his vision of *Homo aquaticus* — an underwater man with lungs and respiratory passages filled with a neutral salt solution replacing air; small oxygenating appendages supplied the body with oxygen by hydrolysis of seawater. In 1968, a scientist exposed mice, their lungs filled with a balanced saline solution, to a pressure of 30 atmospheres. They survived for 18 hours without distress.

Marine mammals (dolphins, seals and whales) may provide interesting clues as to how man could

Champion divers, sperm whales may descend to 10,000 feet and remain there for periods of 90 minutes or so. They can apparently make rapid ascents from such depths without the risks suffered by human divers.

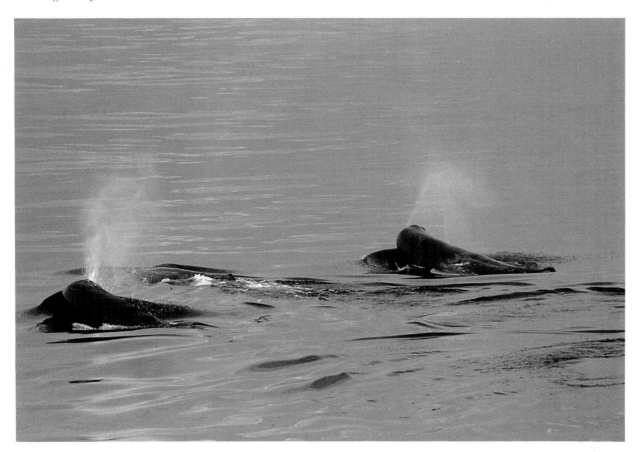

possibly adapt to life underwater. Whales frequently dive for periods of up to 20 minutes and have been known to spend an hour or more at 10,000 feet. There are several physical reasons why whales can survive such long periods of immersion. First, in proportional terms, the metabolic rate of a whale is one-fifteenth that of a human; thus they need relatively less energy and less oxygen. Second, there is a large store of hemoglobin in a whale's muscles that can carry sufficient oxygen to propel the creature at a speed of 5 knots (5¾ miles per hour) for 25 minutes; an even greater oxygen debt would still be tolerated. Third, in common with other aquatic mammals, whales seem to be able to tolerate higher tensions of carbon dioxide in the blood than humans, and their respiratory drive is primarily stimulated by low oxygen levels.

When seals dive, their heart rate decreases from 120 beats a minute at the surface to 4 beats a minute at a depth of 300 feet. While they are submerged,

only vital organs are kept supplied with oxygen. Seals also have specialized blood vessels around the brain and spinal cord which trap bubbles of air and prevent them entering the circulation. Such features demonstrate the enormous adaptability of the basic mammalian respiratory system.

Built to function in a mixture of one-fifth oxygen, four-fifths nitrogen at sea level atmospheric pressure, the human respiratory system is remarkably flexible. Given sufficient time, it adapts to conditions at altitude, making actual physiological changes to enable man to survive. Correct breathing techniques enable athletes to perform their feats, and, with help from breathing apparatus, we can cope with even the most extreme conditions of deep sea and space and make the transition back to normal sea level pressure again. Whatever the situation, oxygen is the prime need of the human body; deprivation for even four minutes can cause brain damage and death.

Appendix

Life-saving Techniques

Many lives have been saved by the common sense and timely intervention of untrained members of the public, when faced with a medical emergency. Many more lives could be saved if certain simple techniques were more widely known: techniques such as the Heimlich maneuver for choking, mouth-to-mouth resuscitation for victims of asphyxia, and cardio-pulmonary resuscitation for cardiac arrest.

Breathing is crucial to the maintenance of life. A four-minute warning alarm is triggered when an accident victim or medical casualty ceases to breathe. If breathing does not recommence and oxygen reach the brain in those four minutes, the brain will be damaged and, shortly after, the patient will die.

A variety of events, such as choking, suffocation, drug overdose, gas poisoning, drowning, electric shock and heart attack, may cause breathing to cease. Other causes are compression of the neck or chest, abrupt change in atmospheric pressure, inhalation of fumes or a severe blow on the head or upper spine sustained, for example, in a road accident.

These and many other incidents may all stop normal respiration. In some, the lungs may remain intact, needing only a moderate forced inflation to get them going again.

Speed is clearly of the

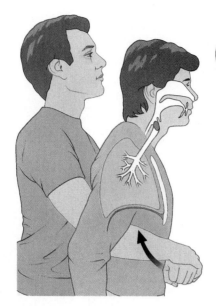

To perform the Heimlich maneuver, stand behind the choking victim with your arms around him just above his navel. Make one hand into a fist, clasp it with the other and thrust up and inward toward the chest.

Each thrust raises the diaphragm and sends a forceful expulsion of air from the lungs to the larynx. Several quick thrusts may be necessary.

If the choking victim collapses, turn her on her back. Kneeling over her, place the heel of one hand above her navel and the other on the back of the first. Give single sharp thrusts down and forward toward the chest.

essence when trying to resuscitate an unconscious victim. Whatever damage has been done to the rest of the body, the chances of survival are zero unless breathing and circulation are restored as quickly as possible. A few breaths of air given by the kiss of life can make the difference between life and death.

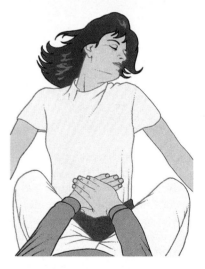

Should you find yourself faced with an emergency in which the victim has stopped breathing, think of the ABC of resuscitation: airways, breathing and circulation. First, clear the airways of any obstruction, such as the tongue, loose or false teeth, blood or vomit. Second, administer mouth-to-mouth resuscitation to force air into, and inflate, the person's lungs.

Third, check the circulation by feeling for the pulse in the carotid artery, the large artery on either side of the neck. If there is no pulse, the heart is probably not beating and cardiopulmonary resuscitation is needed.

Only if you are sure that the heart has stopped beating should you start external heart compression. Place the heel of one hand on the lower half of the sternum and put the other hand on top of the first. If you are alone, do fifteen heart compressions (about one every second) followed by two quick lung inflations by mouth-to-mouth resuscitation. If you have help, do five heart compressions and let your assistant follow with one deep lung inflation. Repeat these sequences continuously until normal breathing is restored.

Choking is a different kind of emergency because once the obstruction has been removed from the airway normal breathing recommences — unless the victim has become unconscious. When something "goes down the wrong way" the simplest means of clearing it is for the victim to cough. If this is not possible, or does not clear the obstruction, there is a real danger of asphyxiation by the blocking piece of food. Often known as a "cafe coronary," because it typically occurs in

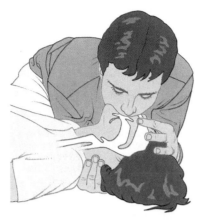

To give mouth-to-mouth resuscitation, open the airway by lifting the victim's neck and tilting back her head. Hold her nose, seal your mouth around hers and blow. Watch for her chest to fall and repeat fifteen times a minute.

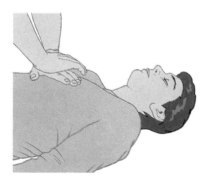

To restart the heart, place the heel of one hand on the lower half of the victim's breastbone and cover it with the heel of the other. Rock forward, pressing firmly down on the bone. Repeat the process at least sixty times a minute.

restaurants, this form of choking often happens when the victim inhales a fibrous item of food such as a lump of meat. The blockage can be so severe that the victim cannot even cry for help.

Before 1974 many people did actually choke to death this way. In that year, however, Dr. Henry Heimlich introduced a means of clearing obstructions from the airway. Known as the Heimlich maneuver this technique has since saved the lives of some 10,000 Americans. Dr. Heimlich has recently received a medical award for his work.

The maneuver involves the rescuer giving sharp thrusts to the abdomen of the victim, forcing the pressure inside the chest cavity to rise and so expel the obstruction.

If you start to choke when alone, you can try the Heimlich maneuver on yourself — with care — but Dr. Heimlich has recently developed an alternative solo version. Raise the chin so that the trachea is straight, and lean over a chairback to administer sudden pressure just below the rib cage. The thrust this provides should clear the obstruction in the same way as the regular maneuver.

All of these techniques must be performed with extreme care and only if there is no alternative action to be taken. Best of all, take a first aid course so that you can act efficiently in any emergency.

Glossary

aerobic the descriptive term for organisms or metabolic activities that require oxygen.

alveolar atelectasis the collapse of alveoli in part of the lung caused by a lack of air. This may occur when a newborn baby's lungs fail to inflate or when part of a lung is blocked.

alveolar capillaries the network of tiny blood vessels that link the pulmonary artery and the pulmonary vein and are involved in gas exchange with the air spaces of the alveoli.

alveolitis inflammation of the alveoli.

alveolus tiny round air spaces in the lungs — the site of gas exchange.

amnesia partial or complete loss of memory.

anaerobic a descriptive term for those organisms which live, and for those metabolisms which proceed, in the absence of oxygen.

analgesia the relief of pain involving the loss of painful impressions without the loss of tactile sense.

anesthesia the loss of sensation brought on either by general anesthetics, which involve the loss of consciousness, or by local anesthetics, which prevent the passage of nervous impulses from a specific region.

angiotensin a potent hormone which, by causing arteries to constrict, increases blood pressure.

aorta the great arterial trunk which rises in an arch from the left ventricle of the heart and sends out its branches to the whole body.

apnea temporary stoppage of breathing brought on when insufficient carbon dioxide in the blood means that the respiratory center in the brain fails to be stimulated.

arteries blood vessels which convey blood away from the heart and to the tissues of the body.

arterioles very small arteries.

artificial respiration the ventilation of the lungs by external means: from the kiss of life to the iron lung.

asbestosis fibrosis of the lungs caused by the inhalation of fine asbestos dust.

asthma a chronic disorder of the lungs, brought on by narrowing of the bronchi and characterized by paroxysms in which breathing is difficult, wheezing occurs and a distressing tightness is felt in the chest.

atmosphere the gaseous envelope which surrounds the earth. The lowest layer contains about 79 percent nitrogen and 21 percent oxygen. One atmosphere is also the standard unit of pressure: 760 mm (29.9 in) of mercury.

atmospheric pressure the pressure exerted by the weight of the air at the surface of the earth.

atria the two upper chambers of the heart, the left atrium and the right atrium, into which blood flows from the veins.

auricles the equivalent of atria in vertebrates other than man.

bends also called decompression sickness, the bends result from sudden reduction in atmospheric pressure, as when divers return from depth to the surface of the water. Nitrogen bubbles out of the blood, collects in the joints and causes the sufferer to bend the joints in an attempt to ease the pain.

bronchiole a tiny branch of a bronchus which terminates in the alveoli of the lung.

bronchitis inflammation of the bronchi involving excessive production of mucus and characterized by coughing, wheezing and varying degrees of breathlessness.

bronchus one of the two tubes into which the trachea divides at its lower end.

capillaries tiny, thin-walled blood vessels which form a network (between, for instance, arterioles and venules) facilitating the rapid exchange of substances between the blood and tissues.

carcinoma malignant growth or cancer.

cardiopulmonary bypass a technique used in open heart surgery whereby the heart and lungs are bypassed by a heart-lung machine. The machine oxygenates the blood and pumps it back into the body. In the meantime the operation is performed on the heart which is empty of blood and has ceased to beat.

carotid arteries the two principal arteries supplying the head with blood, one found on each side of the neck.

cerebrospinal fluid the clear fluid that bathes the brain and the spinal cord; it also fills the ventricles of the brain and the central canal of the spinal cord.

chemoreceptors sensory receptor cells which respond to chemical changes. For example, the receptors in the carotid and aortic bodies detect a fall in the oxygen content of the blood; they automatically trigger an increase in pulmonary ventilation and arterial blood pressure to correct this.

cilia microscopic hairlike projections which line the trachea in their millions and, by their synchronized beating, facilitate the passage of mucus up toward the larynx.

compliance a measure of the stiffness of the chest and/or the lungs. It is a measure of the ease with which lung volume is changed.

coronary circulation the blood supply to and from the tissues of the heart.

corticosteroid a steroid hormone made by the cortex of the adrenal glands or a synthetic member of the same family.

croup an acute inflammation of the upper respiratory tract which results in a paroxysmal cough and noisy inspiration.

dead space the total volume of all the conducting airways of the lung which are not involved in gas exchange, i.e. the trachea, the bronchi and most of the length of the bronchioles. In some pathological conditions this may also include some areas of the alveoli.

dead space ventilation the ventilation of areas of the lung where capillary blood flow has for some reason ceased or become minimal. Such ventilation is wasted since no oxygen can be absorbed and no carbon dioxide removed.

diaphragm   the dome-shaped muscle separating the chest and the abdominal cavities which plays an important part in breathing.

diastole   the relaxation phase of the heart's pumping cycle.

diffuse interstitial fibrosis   the formation of hard fibrous tissue throughout the interstices, or spaces, surrounding the alveoli of the lungs. This leads to loss of elastic recoil and reduced compliance.

diffusion   the passive transfer of gases and other materials across a permeable membrane and along a concentration gradient. For example, the concentrated oxygen in inspired alveolar air diffuses into the blood capillaries where the level of oxygen is low.

dorsal aorta   the main artery in fishes such as sharks, which distributes blood oxygenated in the gills to all parts of the body.

ductus arteriosus   the half-inch long duct, joining the aorta and the pulmonary artery in the fetus, which starts to close at birth.

edema   swelling or puffiness of a tissue caused by retention of excess fluid.

elastic recoil tendency   the tendency of the lungs to be deflated. Under normal conditions this depends on the difference between the pressure in the pleural sac and the alveolar pressure.

embolus   a solid piece of material, such as a blood clot or a fat globule, which circulates in the bloodstream until it becomes lodged in a blood vessel and hinders the flow of blood.

emphysema   a chronic and incurable disorder in which the alveoli are distended and their walls damaged so that the surface area available for gas exchange is reduced.

erythropoietin   a hormone produced by the kidneys that stimulates production of red blood cells in the bone marrow. Its release is triggered by hypoxia.

expiration   the act of breathing air out of the lungs.

expiratory reserve volume   the amount of air which can be forcibly pushed out after a normal exhalation.

Eustachian tube   the canal connecting the middle ear with the nasopharynx. By allowing the air to reach the tympanic cavity, the tube ensures the air pressure is kept even on both sides of the eardrum.

fibrosis   the development of fibrous tissue as a normal healing reaction which occurs in damaged tissue. It involves some scarring, tissue hardening and some loss of normal function. Fibrosis may also be caused by diseases such as pneumoconiosis.

Fick's law   the law applies to the diffusion of a gas across a membrane. The gas will diffuse quicker if the membrane is thin, permeable, of large surface area and is separating a wide difference in gas concentration.

flail chest   the loss of stability of the thoracic cage following a fracture of the sternum and/or ribs.

g-force   the force imposed on anybody or anything that accelerates or decelerates.

gills   the breathing organs of fishes and some larval amphibians. Oxygen-rich water is taken in through the mouth and expelled through the paired gill slits, richly supplied with blood.

glottis   part of the larynx associated with voice production.

granuloma   small masses of cells containing newly formed blood vessels which spring up as a first step in the healing of wounds. Granulomas are caused by such chronic inflammations as occur in TB and syphyllis.

granulomatous   relating to a granuloma.

heart-lung machine   see cardiopulmonary bypass.

Heimlich maneuver   a resuscitation technique used to clear an obstruction of the respiratory airways in a choking victim. It involves giving four forceful compressions upward of the upper abdomen in an attempt to raise the pressure in the thoracic cavity and expel the obstruction.

hemoglobin   the pigment in red blood cells that combines with oxygen, forming oxyhemoglobin, and carries it to all the tissues of the body.

hyperventilation   rapid deep breathing.

hypoventilation   shallow breathing, or underventilation of the lungs

hypoxemia   insufficient oxygen in the arterial blood.

hypoxemic failure   a type of respiratory failure which results from a lack of oxygen in the arterial blood even though carbon dioxide levels are normal.

hypoxia   a lack of oxygen in the body's tissues. Usually used to describe high altitude sickness resulting from breathing rarefied air.

hypoxic drive   at high altitudes, the lack of oxygen in the tissues — hypoxia — takes over from the excess of carbon dioxide in the blood as the main stimulation to breathe.

inspiration   the act of inhaling air into the lungs.

inspiratory reserve volume   the extra air that can be forcibly inhaled after a normal inhalation.

Intensive Care Unit (ICU)   a specialized hospital unit which contains equipment for observing vital body functions and for taking over these functions, such as respiration, should they fail.

intercostal muscles   the twenty-two sets of muscles located between the ribs on each side of the thorax.

intermittent positive pressure ventilation   (IPPV) a technique of artificial respiration in which respirable gases are intermittently forced into the lungs of a patient suffering from respiratory failure. Originally a manual operation, IPPV is now an integral part of life-support systems.

interstitial pulmonary edema   the swelling of the interstitial space around the alveoli due to absorption of water. This leads to reduced gas exchange, reduced lung volumes and loss of compliance.

interstitium   the spaces surrounding the alveoli in the lungs.

interventricular septum   the central wall of the heart which divides it into two and prevents the deoxygenated blood in the right ventricle from mixing with the oxygenated blood in the left ventricle.

Krebs cycle   the series of cyclical metabolic changes by which energy is generated in every cell and oxygen is consumed.

laryngoscope   an instrument for examining the larynx.

larynx   the voice box, lying below the root of the tongue, above the trachea and in front of the lowest part of the pharynx.

lung   the organ of breathing.

meningitis   the bacterial inflammation of the meninges, the membranes surrounding the brain and spinal cord.

mesothelioma   a rapidly fatal tumor, particularly associated with asbestos workers, that spreads over the pleural membrane surrounding the lung.

metastatic   relating to metastasis, the process by which tumor cells break away from a primary site, enter the blood or lymph and set up new colonies elsewhere.

minute volume   the total volume of air moved in each minute of breathing: for the average person, about seven liters.

mitochondria   tiny organelles found in varying numbers in every cell in the body. The powerhouses of the cell, they use oxygen, produce carbon dioxide and generate much of the energy needed by the cell.

molecular weight   the weight of a molecule in comparison with that of a hydrogen atom, which has a molecular weight of 1.

mucus   the viscous fluid secreted by a mucous membrane.

mycoplasma   a group of small organisms intermediate in size between a virus and a bacterium, one of which causes a type of pneumonia.

obstructive lung disease   disease caused by any obstruction, such as sputum or narrowing of the airways, that increases resistance to air flow in the trachea and bronchi.

Ondine's curse   a rare disorder in which breathing is no longer automatic, but is hypoventilatory and subject to pauses.

opioid   any derivative of opium, such as morphine.

organelles   assorted structures, such as mitochondria and ribosomes, found inside cells.

oxidation   the chemical addition of oxygen to something. Hence, carbon is oxidized to carbon dioxide and hydrogen is oxidized to water.

oxidative respiration   the release of energy in the presence of oxygen as found in the Krebs cycle. Such respiration is the main activity of mitochondria.

oxygen tension/concentration   see partial pressure.

oxygenation   the saturation of a substance, particularly blood, with oxygen.

parietal pleura   the pleural membrane lining the inside of the chest wall.

partial pressure   the pressure, or tension, exerted by any one component gas in a gas mixture.

perfusion   the flow of blood into a tissue.

phlogiston   derived from the Greek word meaning inflammable, phlogiston is a hypothetical substance said by many eighteenth-century scientists to be contained in all combustible substances. Burning, like respiration, was thought to release phlogiston into the air.

photosynthesis   the metabolic process by which plants assemble organic molecules, such as carbohydrates, from inorganic ones, such as carbon dioxide and water, using energy from sunlight.

pleura   the thin membranes covering the lungs and the inside of the chest wall.

pleural membrane   the pleura.

pleural sac   the space enclosed by the pleural membranes.

pneuma   air, spirit or breath.

pneumoconiosis   fibrosis of the lung caused by continued inhalation of dust during industrial occupations; particularly associated with coal mining.

pneumonia   inflammation of the lungs caused by bacteria or viruses and characterized by coughing, sweating, chills and fever.

pneumonitis   inflammation of lung tissue.

pneumothorax   the presence of air in the pleural sac, separating the parietal pleura from the visceral pleura, which compresses the lung. A complicated pneumothorax may lead to a collapsed lung.

polyps   small, harmless tumors attached to a mucous membrane by a stalk and occurring in the larynx, nose, cervix or intestines.

premedication   drugs given before the administration of another drug such as an anesthetic. They may be sedatives, such as morphine, or drugs to inhibit the production of saliva and mucus, such as atropine.

prokaryotic   relating to cells, such as those of blue-green algae or bacteria, which do not have a nucleus.

prostaglandins   hormones which are made by a wide variety of body tissues and which have a local effect on smooth muscle.

pulmonary   relating to the lung.

pulmonary arteries   the two blood vessels carrying deoxygenated blood from the right ventricle of the heart, one to each lung.

pulmonary arteriovenous fistula   an opening between a pulmonary artery and its adjacent pulmonary vein that allows blood to be shunted from one to the other.

pulmonary circulation   the blood supply to and from the lungs.

pulmonary edema   an accumulation of fluid in the lungs caused by stagnation of blood in the pulmonary circulation. Brought on by left-sided heart failure or by pulmonary hypertension, it results in breathlessness, especially when lying down.

pulmonary embolism   an obstruction of a pulmonary artery or one of its branches by a large blood clot or by a shower of small emboli.

pulmonary fibrosis   a general term to describe the fibrosis of lung tissue, as may occur in TB, sarcoidosis or interstitial fibrosis.

pulmonary hypertension   a chronic rise in the pressure of blood circulating through the lungs, caused by bronchitis, pulmonary embolism or a number of other disorders.

pulmonary valve   the valve in the heart controlling the flow of blood from the right ventricle into the pulmonary arteries.

pulmonary veins   the two blood vessels, one from each lung, carrying newly oxygenated blood to the left atrium of the heart.

residual volume   the volume of air left in the alveoli and airways after a maximal expiratory effort.

respiratory center   a group of specialized nerve cells in the medulla oblongata at the base of the brain. Spontaneous respiration is completely dependent upon the rhythmic discharge of these cells.

respiratory distress syndrome   a serious disorder affecting the respiration of premature babies who lack the coating of surfactant in their lungs. Breathlessness causes the baby to suffer from hypoxia and cyanosis, and to grunt as it suckles.

restrictive lung disease   the inability to inhale an adequate volume of air compared to normal people of the same height and weight. Restriction may be due to disease in the lung, pleura, chest wall or intercostal muscles.

rete mirabile   from the Latin meaning a miraculous net and referring to a network of fine blood vessels.

sarcoidosis   a rare disorder of the lung in which small areas are inflamed and lymph nodes enlarged. It may lead to fibrosis, pulmonary hypertension and shortness of breath.

shunt   the transfer of blood from one site to another via unusual channels. Shunted blood in the region of the lungs usually returns to the heart without being oxygenated.

silicosis   an incurable disease caused by inhalation of air polluted with silica dust. Particles become lodged in lung tissue and are surrounded irreversibly by scar tissue.

solar plexus   a network of nerve cells and nerve fibers in the abdominal cavity. A part of the autonomic nervous system.

solubility   the ability of a substance to dissolve in water or other solvent.

spirometer   a device for measuring the lung volumes.

sputum   matter, such as mucus, expectorated from the lungs.

sternum   the breastbone.

surface tension   the tendency of liquid surfaces to stick together or to stick to solids. The greater the surface tension of the alveolar fluid, the more likely the alveoli are to collapse.

surfactant   a soapy substance which lowers surface tension. It lines the alveolar membranes and, by reducing their surface tension, prevents the alveoli from collapsing.

systemic arch   the arch of the aorta as it leaves the heart.

systemic circulation   the circulation of blood through the bulk of the body, as opposed to the pulmonary circulation.

systole   the contracting phase of the beating heart, when the ventricular muscles contract and pump blood out of the heart.

tank ventilator   the iron lung, used for artificial respiration in the long-term care of patients with severe weakness in their respiratory muscles.

tendinous   relating to tendons.

thoracic cage   the rib cage.

thoracic cavity   the chest cavity.

thorax   the chest.

thrombus   a blood clot in a blood vessel.

tidal volume   the volume of air that moves into the lungs with each inspiration (or the volume that moves out with each expiration).

total lung capacity   the volume of air contained in the lungs at the end of a maximal inspiration.

trachea   the windpipe, leading from the larynx to the two bronchi.

tracheitis   inflammation of the trachea.

tracheotomy   an operation to facilitate breathing in which a vertical slit is made in the front of the trachea through which a tube is inserted.

tricuspid valve   the valve in the heart which controls the flow of blood from the right atrium into the right ventricle.

tuberculosis   a worldwide endemic disease caused by mycobacteria which often invade the lungs and cause a wasting disease; previously known as consumption.

upper respiratory tract   the nose, the throat, the larynx and the trachea.

vagus   an important nerve which sends branches to the heart, lungs, stomach and other abdominal regions.

vasoconstriction   the narrowing of any blood vessel by the all-round constriction of its walls.

ventilation   breathing in and out.

ventilatory failure   a type of respiratory failure which results from a lack of oxygen and from an excess of carbon dioxide in the blood.

ventricles   the two lower cardiac chambers that receive blood from their respective atria and pump it out of the heart.

visceral pleura   the pleural membrane lining the outside of the lungs.

Illustration Credits

Introduction
6, Science Photo Library.

The Vital Spirit
8, Copyright reserved. Reproduced by gracious permission of Her Majesty The Queen. 10, *Elohim Creating Adam* by William Blake. The Tate Gallery, London. 11, Osterreichische Nationalbibliothek/Bridgeman Art Library. 12, Kim Taylor/Bruce Coleman Limited. 13, Bildarchiv Preussischer Kulturbesitz. 14, *The Challenge in the Wilderness* by Edward Burne-Jones. By courtesy of Christies/Bridgeman Art Library. 15, Mary Evans Picture Library. 16, (left) Mansell Collection, (right) Mary Evans Picture Library. 17, *The Triumph of St. Thomas Aquinas* (detail) by Benozzo Gozzoli. Louvre/ Bulloz. 18, (left) Archiv für Kunst und Geschichte, (right) **Michael McGuinness**. 19, Ann Ronan Picture Library. 20, Mansell Collection. 21, National Library of Medicine. 22, (left) Ann Ronan Picture Library, (right) By courtesy of the National Portrait Gallery, London. 23, By courtesy of the New York Historical Society/Mansell Collection.

The Developing System
24, Howard Sochurek/The John Hillelson Agency. 26, **Michael Courtney**. 27, Camerapix Hutchison Library. 28, (top) **Les Smith**, (bottom) John Watney Photo Library. 29, Zefa UK Limited. 30, Mansell Collection. 31, (top) Herwarth Voigtmann/Planet Earth Pictures, (bottom) Hans Reinhard/Bruce Coleman Limited. 32, (top) Udo Hirsch/Bruce Coleman Limited, (bottom) Hans Reinhard/Bruce Coleman Limited. 33, **Michael Courtney**. 34, G.D. Plage/Bruce Coleman Limited. 35, Joe Baker/The Image Bank. 36, **Michael Courtney**. 37, Anthea Sieveking/Zefa UK Limited.

The Mechanics of Breathing
38, *Dance Marathon* by Phillip Evergood. James and Mari Michener Collection, Archer M. Huntington Art Gallery, The University of Texas at Austin. 40, (top) Michael Abbey/ Science Photo Library, (bottom) Gower Medical Publishing Limited. 41, **Michael Courtney**. 42, (top) Dr. Tony Brain/Science Photo Library, (bottom) John Watney Library. 43, Mansell Collection. 44-5, **Michael Courtney**. 46, Dr. G. Settles/Science Photo Library. 47, John Watney Photo Library. 48-9, **Frank Kennard**. 50, **Les Smith**. 51, John Watney Photo Library. 52, K.R. Porter/Science Photo Library. 53, **Michael Courtney**. 54, Eric Bouvet/

Frank Spooner Pictures. 55, John Watney Photo Library. 56, Science Photo Library. 58, Professor J.B. West. 59, Ann Ronan Picture Library.

Faulty Airways
60, *L'hôtel des Roches Noires à Trouville* by Claude Monet. Jeu de Paume/ Réunion des Musées Nationaux. 62, *Le lit* by Henri Toulouse-Lautrec. Jeu de Paume/Réunion des Musées Nationaux. 63, Kobal Collection. 64, Mansell Collection. 65, American Lung Association. 66, **Michael Courtney**. 67, Ann Ronan Picture Library. 68, (top) Ann Ronan Picture Library, (bottom) **Les Smith**. 69, **Les Smith**. 70, John Watney Photo Library. 71, (top) **Les Smith**, (bottom) **Michael Courtney**.

Disorders of the Lungs
Le Fumeur by Joos van Craesbeeck. Louvre/ Réunion des Musées Nationaux. 74, Ann Ronan Picture Library. 75, (top) Ann Ronan Picture Library, (bottom) **Michael Courtney**. 76, BBC Hulton Picture Library. 77, Gower Medical Publishing Limited. 78, American Cancer Society. 79, Stuart Franklin/Sygma/The John Hillelson Agency. 80, Kobal Collection. 81, (left) John Watney Photo Library, (right) American Cancer Society. 82, John Watney Photo Library. 83, Division of Computer Research and Technology/National Institutes of Health/Science Photo Library. 84, (left) Bibliothèque Nationale/Bulloz, (right) Dr. R. Dourmashkin/Science Photo Library. 85, Centers for Disease Control, Atlanta. 86, Mary Evans Picture Library. 87, Bildarchiv Preussischer Kulturbesitz. 88, (top) John Watney Photo Library, (bottom) Department of Medical Illustration, St. Bartholomew's Hospital, London. 89, Archiv für Kunst und Geschichte. 90, Burt Glinn/Magnum/The John Hillelson Agency. 91, (left) John Watney Photo Library, (right) Department of Medical Illustration, St. Bartholomew's Hospital, London. 92, Henry Gruyaert/ Magnum/The John Hillelson Agency. 93, (left) Gower Medical Publishing Limited, (right) Department of Medical Illustration, St. Bartholomew's Hospital, London. 94, Paul Fusco/Magnum/The John Hillelson Agency. 95, Ian Berry/Magnum/The John Hillelson Agency. 96, (top) Bamberger/ Frank Spooner Pictures, (bottom) Tim Bieber/The Image Bank. 97, (left) *Haymaking – July* (detail) by Pieter Bruegel. National Gallery, Prague/Bridgeman Art Library, (right) Bettman Archive/BBC Hulton Picture Library. 99, (top) John Watney Photo Library, (bottom) National Heart, Lung and Blood Institute/National Institutes of Health. 100, W. von dem Bussche/The Image Bank. 101, General Electric Company Inc. 102, American

Cancer Society. 103, Will McIntyre/Science Photo Library.

Technology Takes Over
104, Francis A. Countway Library of Medicine, Massachussetts. 106, Mansell Collection. 107, Mary Evans Picture Library. 108, Mansell Collection. 109, Wellcome Institute Library, London. 110, Professor M.K. Sykes/Nuffield Department of Anaesthetics, Oxford. 111, John Wright/Camerapix Hutchison Library. 112, *The Lifeline* by Winslow Homer. Philadelphia Museum of Art. George W. Elkins Collection. 113, Mary Evans Picture Library. 114, Guido A. Rossi/The Image Bank. 115, Hans Schmied/Zefa UK Limited. 116, Zefa UK Limited. 118, **Les Smith**.

Breathing Under Pressure
120, *Football* (1917) by Robert Delaunay. Musée d'Art Moderne, Troyes. 122, **Les Smith**. 123, Archiv für Kunst und Geschichte. 124, Kobal Collection. 125, Chris Bonington/Bruce Coleman Limited. 126-7, John Cleare/Mountain Camera. 128, (left) John Cleare/Mountain Camera, (right) Chris Bonington/Bruce Coleman Limited. 129-31, NASA/Science Photo Library. 132, Morton Beebe/The Image Bank. 133, Mansell Collection. 134, **Les Smith**. 135, Alex Hubrich/The Image Bank. 136, Nicholas Devore/Bruce Coleman Limited. 137, Camilla Jessel. 138, Christopher Cormack. 139, Thomas Neerken/Frank Spooner Pictures. 140, **Les Smith**. 141, Peter Scoones/Planet Earth Pictures. 142, Petit Palais/Bulloz. 143, Mansell Collection. 144, Mike Coltman/ Planet Earth Pictures. 145, Ann Ronan Picture Library. 146, **Les Smith**. 147, Dick Clarke/Planet Earth Pictures. 148, Flip Schulke/Planet Earth Pictures. 149, Francisco Erize/Bruce Coleman Limited.

Appendix
150–51, **Les Smith**

Index

heparin, 117
hiccup, 29
Histoplasma capsulatum, 88
histoplasmosis, 88
Hooke, Robert, 21, **22**
humors, four, 16–17
hydrocarbons, 95, **95**
hyperventilation, 126
hypoventilation, 60–61, 63, 64
hypoxemia, 57, 59, 63, 119, 139
hypoxic drive, 126
hypoxic failure, 119

I
Ibu al-Nafis, 19, 20
infections, 84–90
  see also colds, influenza,
    pneumonia, tuberculosis
influenza, 84, **84**
inspiratory mechanism, 28
intensive care, 119
interstitial fibrosis, 70
iron lung, 114

J
Jackson, Charles, 106, 107

K
Kartagener's syndrome, 80
kidneys, 44
Koch, Robert, 89
Krebs cycle, 134
kyphoscoliosis, 63, **63**

L
laryngoscope, 116
larynx, 40, **41**
Lavoisier, Antoine, 39, 43, 119
Legionnaire's disease, 85, **85**
life-support machines, 114
lipids, 47
Lister, Robert, 107
liver, 18
Lowe, Richard, 21
lungs, in blood flow, 19–20, 59
  cancer, 80–84, **81**
  collapse, 70
  disease types, 68–69
  and exercise, 132–34
  fetal development, 34, **34**, 36, **36**, 37
  function, 14–15, 26–28, 29, 39, 44, 50,
    51, 59
  function in animals, 32–33
  infection in tuberculosis, 87, **88**
  inhalation diseases, 90–98
    see also pneumoconiosis,
      asbestosis, silicosis
  malfunctions, 61–71
  obstructive disease, 69–70
  physiology, 13–14, 40, **42**, **54**, 69–70

in pulmonary embolism, 98
  tissue break down, 76
  volume, 50, 69, 70–71
lungfish, 31–32
lymph nodes in tuberculosis, 87

M
Malpighi, Marcello, 21, **21**
Mayow, John, 21
mesothelioma, 84, 93, 95
mitochondria, 13
morphine, 105
Morton, William, 106, 107, **108**
mountain sickness, 127–29
mucus, 39, 42, **42**, 69, 75
muscle, intercostal, 28
  relaxants, 111–13
Mycobacterium tuberculosis, 87

N
narcotics, 62
nasal cavity, 39–40
nitrogen, 11, 144, 146, **146**
nitrous oxide, 106, **106**, 107
nostrils, 39
nuclear magnetic resonance, 102

O
oat cell carcinoma, 81, 82
obesity, 64, 71
obstructive lung disease, 69–70
Ondine's curse, 63
opium, 105
oxygen, and altitude, 121, 124, 126, 129
  in atmosphere, 121–22
  in blood flow, 10, 11, 22, 25, 39, **39**,
    43, 44, **44**, 122
  diffusion of, 51–53, 65
  and exercise, 132–34, 137–38
  reduced supply, 61–62, 67, 68, 76,
    114
  supply in animals, 32–33
  volume inhaled, 50
oxygenator, in bypass surgery, 117–18

P
penicillin, 85
phlogiston theory, 22–23, 43
photosynthesis, 11, 13, **13**, **27**
Pickwickian syndrome, 64, **64**
"pink puffers," 76
placenta, 37
pleural diseases, 70–71
pleural membrane, 39
pleural sac, 28
"pneuma," 16–17, 18
pneumoconiosis, 90, **90**
pneumonia, 67, 84–85
pneumonitis, 97
pneumothorax, 70–71, **70**

polio, 63
pollution, of air, 90, 95–97, **95**, **96**
"premedication," 115, 117
Priestley, Joseph, 22, 23, **23**, 43
prokaryotic organisms, 11
"psyche," 17
pulmonary arteries, 19, 21, 36, 54, 56,
  56, 98
pulmonary arteriovenous fistula, 67
pulmonary edema, 67, 99, **99**, 128–29,
  128
pulmonary embolism, 67, 98
pulmonary hypertension, 98
pulmonary sequestrations, 73

R
Raleigh, Sir Walter, 111
reptiles, 33
respiration, scientific discovery of,
  14–15
respiratory distress syndrome (RDS),
  47, **47**
respiratory failure, 118–19
respiratory rate, 57
resuscitation, 114, 150–51
rheumatoid arthritis, 102
rib cage, 26–28, 39

S
sarcoidosis, 70, 102
scuba diving, 142–44, **141**
seals, 149
septum, 18
Servetus, Miguel, 19–20
sharks, 30–31, **31**
silicosis, 86, 90, **91**
Simpson, James, 106, 109
sleep, effect on respiration, 62, **63**
sneezing, 29, **29**
Snow, John, 108, 109
space travel, effect on respiration,
  129–32
spirometry, 50, **50**
sputum, 76, 85
squamous cell carcinoma, 81, 82
sternum, 28
Streptococcus pneumoniae, 84
surfactant, 37, 47
systole, 53, 54

T
Thermophilic actinomycetes, 97
thiopental, 110–11, 116
thoracic volume, enlargement of, 63–64
thorax, 63, 109
trachea, 15, 29, 40, **40**
  in artificial ventilation, 115
  obstruction of, 74
tracheitis, 42
tracheotomy, 113

Printed in Belgium